Inspection of Face and Body for Diagnosis of Diseases

Chief Compiler: Liu Bangming
Translator: Wang Tai

FOREIGN LANGUAGES PRESS BEIJING

First Edition 2002

Home Page:
http://www.flp.com.cn
E-mail Addresses:
info@flp.com.cn
sales@flp.com.cn

ISBN 7-119-02028
©Foreign Languages Press, Beijing, China, 2002
Published by Foreign Languages Press
24 Baiwanzhuang Road, Beijing 100037, China
Distributed by China International Book Trading Corporation
35 Chegongzhuang Xilu, Beijing 100044, China
P. O. Box 399, Beijing, China
Printed in the People's Republic of China

CONTENTS

Chapter 1
DIAGNOSIS OF DISEASES BY INSPECTION OF FACIAL FEATURES

Can a diagnosis of disease be made by inspecting the facial features of a patient?

According to the theories of medicine and genetics, the facial features of human beings can show the health condition of the human body and provide information about diseases. In the clinical practice of both traditional Chinese and Western medicine, the inspection of facial features has been used as an important diagnostic method for thousands of years.

Following the rapid development of genetic engineering and chromosome technology in recent years, abnormalities in the facial features and bodily constitution of patients with hereditary diseases have increasingly attracted the attention of medical scientists all over the world, and many useful experiences in observing the physique, limbs, sense organs, hair and skin of patients have been accumulated through clinical practice. This has further provided scientific evidence for the application of inspection of facial features in clinical diagnosis of diseases.

I. Inspection of the Head and Diagnosis of Diseases

The head is the top part of the human body, and the brain

in the head is the most important organ controlling all other parts of body, as well as the mental activities. It is also an organ to which all Yang qi scattered in the body may assemble together. Therefore, the observation of the shape, posture and movement of the head, and the color, luster and appearance of the hair can provide information on diseases of the brain and kidneys, and indicate excessiveness or deficiency of qi and blood.

1. The shape of the head: As proposed by ancient raditional Chinese physicians:

1) People with big skulls tend to live longer than those with small skulls.

2) People with wide faces, broad foreheads, regular facial features and thick earlobes tend to have long lives, and their diseases are easily curable; but persons with narrow faces, disarranged sense organs and small and thin earlobes tend to die at an early age.

3) An over-large head in a child may be caused by congenital hydrocephalus; an extra-small head indicates physical underdevelopment of children or deficiency of kidney essence; a bulging fontanel indicates brain and spinal cord disease; retarded closure of the fontanel is a result of poor congenital endowment or deficiency of kidney qi; the premature closure of the fontanel in a case of microcephaly with small and narrow vertex of the head, low forehead and poor intelligence may be due to congenital deficiency of essence.

4) A weak neck with difficulty supporting the head is due to deficiency of qi, blood and kidney qi.

5) A stiff neck is caused by excessiveness of pathogens in the body; and a drooped head or head inclined to one side is

due to deficiency of vital energy.

2. Posture and movement of the head:

The circumference of the head is a criterion for estimating the normality of development of the brain in children, and it may be affected by endocrinal and metabolic disturbance.

1) Measurement of cranial circumference: A tape measure is used to measure the circumference of the head through the external occipital tuberosity.

2) Normal cranial circumference: The normal value of cranial circumference is 34 cm in newborn babies; 42 cm in babies of 6 months; 45 cm in babies of 1 year; 48 cm in babies of 2 years; 50 cm in children of 4 years; and 51 cm in children of 10 years. After that, the increase of cranial circumference gradually slows down until 18 years of age, with an average value of 51-53 cm in adult men and 50-57 cm in adult women.

3) Extra-large cranial circumference or abnormally rapid increase of cranial circumference: This may occur in children with rickets, macrocephaly, lesions occupying intracranial space, chronic subdural hematoma, hydrocephalus, cretinism, megalencephlon, vitamin A poisoning or vitamin A deficiency; and it may also appear in adults with acromegaly, subgaleal hematoma and osteitis deformans.

4) Extra-small cranial circumference: This may occur in cases of true microcephaly, such as familial hereditary microcephaly (acrocephaly) with a circumference of less than 43 cm or even as small as 25 cm; and it may also appear in acquired intracranial diseases, such as underdevelopment or atrophy of the brain caused by inflammation, external trauma or premature closure of fontanel.

5) Declination of the head: Forward declination of the head

may be caused by deficiency of Zhong qi (qi of the middle energizer) in patients with sallow complexion, weakness of the body, mental tiredness and shortness of breath; or it may be caused by deficiency of brain material in patients with tinnitus, deafness, and soreness and weakness of the waist and knees.

6) Posture of head with chin up: The opisthotonus posture of head with the chin up and eyes staring upward may occur in patients with tetanus or acute convulsions.

7) Inclination of the head: Inclination of the head to one side with limitation of movement may appear in patients with acute sprain.

8) Tremor of the head: Tremor of the head may be caused by upward attack of Yang wind pathogens or stirring up of endogenous deficient wind pathogens.

9) Abnormal movement of the head: Limitation of movement of the head may occur in patients with cervical spondylosis; tremor of the head may appear in Parkinson's disease patients; the nodding-head movement keeping pace with the pulsation of the carotid artery is a symptom of severe aortic insufficiency; and fixed head without any movement is caused by cervical spondylitis.

II. Inspection of Abnormal Facial Features

1) Senile face: The face looks much older than the actual age of the patient in cases of senilism, congenital general lipo-atrophy, dwarfism with deafness or lipo-atrophic diabetes mellitus.

2) Contorted face: Contorted face may occur in patients with acrocephalosyndactyly.

3) Dull face: The disarrangement of the sense organs and dull facial expression may occur in patients with mongolism or microphthalmia with mental retardation.

4) Widely separated eyes: Widely separated eyes may accompany more than 30 kinds of diseases, including absence of the short arm of chromosome 4, mongolism and hypoplasia of cranial and facial bones.

5) Upward-directed outer canthus of the eye: Both the outer canthi of the eyes are abnormally directed upward in patients with mongolism or congenital localized keratoconus.

6) Downward-inclined outer canthus of the eye: Both outer canthi of the eyes are abnormally inclined downward in patients with congenital obese dysplasia, imperfect osteogenesis of the mandibular, cranial and facial bones, multiple deformities of facial bones or mongolism.

7) Microphthalmia: The eyeballs are hidden behind extraordinarily narrow eye fissures in patients with cryptophthalmia, congenital panhematopenia or congenital obese dysplasia.

8) Ophthalmos: The eyeballs protrude in patients with neurofibroma, arteriovenous aneurysm of the retina, general petrification of bones or hereditary amyloidosis of nerves.

9) Broad nose bridge: The nose bridge is low, flat, broad and almost saddle-shaped in patients with mongolism or multiple basal cell nevi.

10) Cleft lip and palate: The cleft lip (hare lip) and cleft palate (wolf throat) may occur in patients with trisomy 13 syndrome, joint-brain-palate dysplasia or congenital dysplasia of the testis.

11) Extra small skull: The fontanels of babies are usually closed by the age of 12-18 months. If they are prematurely closed, the babies may develop microcephaly with mental

retardation.

12) Sharp skull: Because of the premature closure of fontanels and cranial fissures, babies may develop a small head with a narrow forehead and a sharp vertex of the skull; this is a common deformity of microcephaly.

13) Square skull: Babies suffering from rickets or congenital syphilis may develop a square skull with protruded frontal tubers and flattened vertex of the head.

14) Boat-like skull: Because of the premature closure of the sagital fissure of the skull babies suffering from microcephaly may develop a boat-like skull due to the expansion of the skull to the anterior side.

15) Flat skull: This condition may occur in babies with congenital microcephaly or mongolism.

16) Deformed skull: This condition appears in middle-aged people, involving an enlarged skull and thickened bony matrix with curved long bones.

17) Small lower jaw: Babies suffering from micrognathia, cat-cry syndrome or multiple facial deformities may develop an apparently small and backward-retracted jaw.

III. Bodily Features and Susceptible Diseases

Different types of bodily features (Fig. 1-1).

1) Respiratory type: People of this type may have a bulging and fusiform face, prominent cheekbones, pigeon chest, slender backbone, reverse ladder-shaped trunk, rounded chin and narrow pupil distance. They have well developed respiratory organs and good pulmonary function, but some of them may suffer from chronic diseases of the throat and a high sus-

ceptibility to diseases of the respiratory system.

2) Digestive type: People of this type may have a pyramid-shaped face with thick soft tissue and muscles around the lower part of face, big mouth, thick lips and protruding belly. This is a bodily feature type derived from the respiratory type, when ancient people migrated out of the forests and began to live on the plains. They are susceptible to diarrhea.

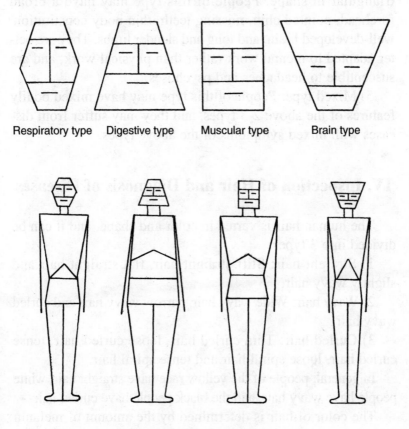

Respiratory type　　Digestive type　　Muscular type　　Brain type

Fig. 1-1　Different types of bodily features

3) Muscular type: People of this type may have a well- proportional face and body, barrel-shaped trunk, long limbs and well-developed muscles and bones. The nose bridge is not very high, and the chin is not very pointed. The forehead is high, broad and square in shape. They are susceptible to arthritis and muscle ache.

4) Brain type: The skull is well developed and the face is triangular in shape. People of this type may have a broad forehead, pointed chin, missing teeth, thin body constitution, well-developed brain, and long and slender limbs. They are better adapted to mental work rather than physical work, and are susceptible to headaches and psychoses.

5) Mixed type: People of this type may have mixed bodily features of the above 2-3 types, and they may suffer from diseases with mixed symptoms of the above types.

IV. Inspection of Hair and Diagnosis of Diseases

The human hair is varied in color and shape, and it can be divided into 3 types:

1) Straight hair: Stiff straight hair, flat straight hair and slightly wavy hair.

2) Wavy hair: Wide wavy hair, narrow wavy hair and curled wavy hair.

3) Curled hair: Thin curled hair, loose curled hair, tense curled hair, loose spiral hair and tense spiral hair.

In general, people of the yellow race have straight hair, white people have wavy hair, and the black people have curled hair.

The color of hair is determined by the amount of melanin (black pigment) in it. The hair may be blacker in color if it contains more granular melanin pigment; the hair may be red in color if it contains soluble melanin pigment; and the hair may be blond in color if it contains much soluble melanin pigment. In general, Chinese people have black or dark-brown hair.

Hair tends to turn gray with age. From middle age, the vesicles in the hair increase in number, and the granules of black pigment decreased in amount. The hair may therefore turn brown, and hair with air in the vesicles may turn white.

The color of hair, skin and eyes is determined by the amount of melanin in them, and their color in an individual is mutually matched and correlated.

The length of hair is related to its shape. Straight hair may grow over 1 meter in length; curled hair is usually very short; and the length of wavy hair is in-between. Within the same race, the hair of women may grow longer than that of men, and the difference between the sexes is more remarkable in people with wavy hair.

Hair may grow 0.3 mm in one day and night. The stiffness of hair is closely related to its thickness, and its density is also related to its thickness. The total number of hairs in an individual is about 100 thousand.

According to traditional Chinese medical theory, the condition of hair is dependant of the state of the blood, and it can reveal the condition of the kidneys. Therefore, people with plentiful blood and kidney qi tend to have black and lustrous hair.

(1) *Pathological hair:*

1) Presenile grey hair in young people, together with dizziness and tinnitus, as well as soreness and weakness in the waist and legs, is caused by deficiency of kidney qi; and pres-

enile grey hair in young people, together with symptoms of deficiency of heart qi is due to mental fatigue and depletion of blood.

2) Generalized grey hair is caused by albinism; and localized white hair is due to vertiligo.

3) Temporary occurrence of much grey hair in people with bad temper, annoyance, flushing face and bitter taste in the mouth is caused by accumulation of heat pathogens in the liver.

4) Yellow hair is caused by deficiency of blood or is due to heat pathogens in qi and blood.

5) Yellow, sparse and dry hair is caused by deficiency of blood and essence; and yellow and dry hair in people with a wan and sallow complexion is due to chronic disease, weakness of the body and malnutrition.

6) Straight dry hair is caused by depletion of qi and body fluid; and wet hair due to constant spontaneous sweating in patients with shortness of breath is caused by exhaustion of the lungs.

7) Sparse, thin and soft hair especially remarkable over the vertex and temporal region of head in patients with vertigo, soreness and weakness of the waist and knees, tidal fever and emission of semen is due to deficiency of blood and essence.

8) Sparse hair with itching and desquamation of the scalp is due to seborrheic dermatitis.

9) Loss of hair may be caused by diseases due to attack of wind pathogens, dryness pathogens in the blood, seborrheic dermatitis, alopecia areata, typhoid fever, leprosy, cirrhosis of the liver or malignant tumors.

10) Tangled hair with extremely lean body and distended abdomen may occur in children suffering from indigestive malnutrition.

10

(2) *Loss of hair:*

Loss of hair is caused by the mutation of genes. Loss of hair in patches is due to deficiency of Yin and blood in the liver and kidneys, failure of communication between the heart and the kidneys, and invasion of external wind pathogens into a deficient body.

1) Loss of hair in patches: Hair may be lost in one or several patches with regular margin and normal skin. It may occur in patients of alopecia areata or leprosy.

2) Total baldness: The hair over the whole scalp may be completely lost within a short period of time, and it may be gradually caused by the progression of alopecia areata. The skin of the scalp is normal. It may occur in aged people or patients of late-stage typhoid fever.

3) Premature baldness: From the late stage of the prime of life, the gradual loss of hair starts from the corners of the forehead, and then spreads over the vertex to the occipital region of the head, with the hair over the peripheral region of the scalp remaining normal.

4) Diffuse loss of hair: Diffuse loss of hair is caused by acute infectious diseases, chronic diseases or intoxication due to chemicals or drugs.

5) Congenital baldness: This is a dominant genetic disease of the chromosomes occurring in successive generations of a family.

6) False alopecia areata: In middle-aged men, hair may be lost in one or 2 small round patches with clear margins, and then the bare patches may gradually increase in size and fuse together. The local smooth and shiny skin may become atrophic, thinner and depressed. The hair loss may stop spontaneously, but the lost hair can not be regenerated.

7) Postpartum loss of hair: The hair may be gradually lost in women 2-5 months after delivery of a baby, and it may continue for 2-6 months.

8) Loss of hair due to endocrinal diseases: The hair may turn dry, fragile, sparse, thicker or thinner in patients with hyperthyroidism, hypothyroidism, hypoparathyroidism or diseases of the pituitary gland.

9) Peripheral baldness: The hair on the peripheral region of the scalp may be lost, with uneven and sparse hair preserved.

10) Loss of hair around the nevus: The hair around the pigmented nevus on the scalp may be lost, leaving local baldness as a lesion of alopecia areata.

11) Circular baldness: The hair may be lost, leaving a circular naked patch.

(3) *Scalp dandruff:*
Scalp dandruff is the small fine scales detached from the scalp. The formation of excess dandruff is related to heredity and mental agitation.

Chapter 2
INSPECTION OF THE FACE AND DIAGNOSIS OF DISEASES

The face is a comprehensive display window of the human body.

According to Chen Shiduo, a traditional physician of the Qing Dynasty: "The color of various parts of the face must be carefully observed when making diagnosis of diseases." Abnormal changes of the color and luster of the face should be carefully observed. Different colors displayed in the face may show different diseases in the body; and the change of luster can reflect the richness of essence in the body.

I. Normal and Abnormal Facial Color and Diagnosis of Diseases

As people of the yellow race, Chinese persons normally have faces with mixed red and yellow colors, with a gentle and soft brightness to indicate that they have rich stomach qi and good spirits. The good spirits in an individual can be shown by a shiny face, and rich stomach qi can be shown by a faint yellow complexion. Because of the variation of the bodily constitution in human beings, people may have modified facial colors, with red, black, white or yellow tinges; at the same time, the change of physiological condition may also produce a modification of facial color to show red, blue or white tints. However, these are all in the normal range of facial color. The facial color can be divided into the basic color and modified color.

(1) *Basic facial color:*
Facial color is varied from race to race. As a branch of the yellow race, the Chinese people have a light yellow facial color. This is the basic facial color of Chinese people, although it may be slightly modified in people with different hereditary characteristics, life style, job, sex and age.

(2) *Modified facial color:*
The physiological functions of human beings are closely related to the change of environment. The facial color may be slightly modified by the change of seasons as well as the change of time in the day. For example, the facial color may be slightly blue in spring, slightly red in summer, slightly white in autumn and slightly black in winter; and the complexion is brighter during the day, because qi travels through Yang meridians, and it is slightly dim at night as qi passes through Yin meridians. The facial color can also be affected by living conditions, life style and social environment. Emotional disturbance may also apparently change the facial color. For example, the face may flush with shame, or turn pale and dull with worry and sadness; an angry person may display a red face, but it may turn yellowish white in a person with prolonged fury; and a happy person may have a radiant and pleasant face. The facial color can also be changed by tiredness or relaxation, quality of sleep, fullness or emptiness of the stomach and the intake of alcohol.

14

However, the change of facial color caused by the above factors is a temporary fluctuation limited within the normal range, and it is therefore called modified facial color.

(3) *Pathological facial color:*

This is the facial color of patients suffering from various diseases. The abnormal facial color of patients can show the specific pathological disturbance in the internal organs of the body. It can be divided into benign pathological color with a vague brightness and malignant pathological color with a wan, sallow and haggard appearance.

The benign color indicates a better prognosis, with the internal organs not badly damaged and much vital energy still preserved; but the malignant color indicates a bad prognosis with at least one internal organ badly damaged, and stomach qi exhausted or the essence almost depleted. Therefore, it is also called a "dying color." Under certain conditions, the benign and malignant facial colors can be mutually exchanged, and the developmental trend of a disease can be predicted from the exchange of benign and malignant colors. The change of facial color from benign type to malignant type indicates the aggravation of a disease, and conversely it indicates the alleviation of a disease.

In addition, the coincidence of facial color with the nature of a disease is also an index for making a prognosis of a disease. If the facial color matches the nature of the disease, it is called the ordinary facial color of the disease, otherwise it is an extraordinary facial color of the disease. For example, the face of a patient with a liver disease should be blue, which is the ordinary facial color of liver diseases. According to the Theory of the Five Elements, the five colors (red, blue, yellow, white and black) can mutually promote or counteract. In patients with liver diseases, a yellow facial color indicates a bad prognosis, and a white facial color indicates aggravation of the diseases.

The face of patients may often show a mixed color, rather than a pure color, and the fractions of color may be distributed in different areas of the face or mixed up to form an even color. For example, a white color may mix with black, yellow, blue or red colors.

When inspecting the facial color, the depth, clearness, darkness, distribution and brightness of the color should be carefully observed.

The color of the face may be exposed on the superficial skin or penetrate deeply into the tissue. The superficial color indicates a disease in the superficial structures of the body or in the hollow internal organs; and a color which has penetrated deeply into the tissues indicates a disease in the deep structures of the body or in the solid internal organs. The change of depth of facial color may show the spread of disease between different structures and internal organs. The facial color may be clear or turbid. A clear color indicates a disease in Yang (meridians, structures or organs) and the turbid color indicates a disease in Yin (meridians, structures or organs); and the change of clearness of color may show the spread of disease between Yin and Yang. A light facial color indicates excessiveness of vital energy (body resistance) and a dark color indicates excessiveness of pathogens in the body. The change of depth of color may show the change of dominance of body resistance or pathogens. Scattered color over the face indicates the alleviation of disease, concentrated color indicates the aggravation of disease, and the change of distribution of facial color can show the development of disease. A bright facial color indicates intact qi and blood, and a dull color indicates loss of spirit. The change of brightness of facial color can show the developmental tendency of a disease.

II. Facial Colors and Diagnosis of Diseases

According to the Theory of the Five Elements, the five facial colors (red, blue, yellow, white and black) are the representative colors of the five internal organs, respectively.

How does one diagnose diseases in the different organs from the five facial colors? Blue color is related to wind pathogens and liver diseases; red color is related to heat pathogen and heart diseases; yellow color is related to dampness pathogens and spleen diseases; white color is related to cold pathogens and lung diseases; and black color is related to infectious pathogens and kidney diseases.

(1) *Red color:*
Red facial color is due to engorgement of cutaneous blood vessels in the face of patients with diseases caused by heat pathogens. Dark red is due to attack of excessive heat pathogens, and pale red color is due to attack of deficient heat pathogens.

The flushed face, as seen in a drunken person, is due to heat pathogens in the stomach, The red cheeks of chronic patients appearing in the afternoon is due to attack of deficient heat pathogens. A red color all over the face is due to excessiveness of Yang qi or attack of excessive heat pathogens. Wandering pink color in the cheeks may occur in chronic or critical patients with cold hands and feet. Fresh red color on the whole face with profuse sweating is caused by attack of summer heat pathogens. Red cheeks with dry lips appearing in the afternoon is due to deficiency of Yin and excessiveness of fire pathogens. A red face with sad look and no redness in the eyes is due to sorrow and worry. A red face with a tired look and red eyes is due to insomnia. Purplish red cheeks and lips may occur in patients with rheumatic or coronary heart disease. A bright red face is due to heat pathogens accumulated in the upper part of the body and cold pathogens in the lower part. A dull red face is due to heat pathogens in the lower part of the body and cold pathogens in the upper part. A red face with tidal fever and delirium is due to accumulation of excessive heat pathogens in the hollow organs. Coughing with yellow sputum in patients with red face and dry throat is caused by heat pathogen. Red color appearing around the nose with much seborrheic excretion is a physical sign of acne rosacea (brandy nose). A butterfly-like erythema beside the nose and on the cheeks is a physical sign of lupus erythematosus. In patients of lung diseases, the red facial color resists treatment. A flushed face and ears after sports, bathing, emotional excitement, drinking alcoholic beverages or shame is a normal physiological response.

(2) *Blue color:*

Blue facial color is usually related to diseases of the liver and gallbladder, and diseases with pain or caused by cold and wind pathogens. The blue color is caused by the contraction of capillary blood vessels of the skin, and blockage of qi and blood in meridians.

Blue facial color may appear in patients with diseases of the liver and gallbladder; a blue face with red cheeks is due to malaria with chills and fever or febrile diseases with pain; a dark blue face and eyes, with sudden aphasia, weakness of limbs and difficulty standing up are due to attack of deficient cold pathogens into the liver; a blue face with anger, pain in the flanks and dry throat is due to attack of excessive wind pathogens into the liver; a pale blue color in the eyes with mental depression, numbness and pain of fingers and muscular spasm in the legs is due to attack of deficient wind pathogens into the liver; a blackish-blue facial color is due to severe pain caused by violent cold pathogens; a blue bulb of the nose is due to abdominal pain caused by cold pathogens; a pale blue face is due to severe pain or shock; a greenish blue facial color is due to exhaustion of liver qi; a greyish blue facial color with cyanotic lips is due to deficiency of heart Yang or stasis of heart blood; a dull or dark blue facial color in patients with diseases of any duration is due to deficiency of Yang qi; the facial color is blue or dim blue in patients with chronic liver diseases; the facial color is pure blue in patients with diseases of the spleen and stomach; the sudden appearance of blue facial color in normal subjects is due to fright and fear; a blue color may appear over the nose bridge, between the eyebrows and around the mouth as a prodromal sign of convulsions in children with high fever; in women, a blue facial color and red cheeks indicates Shaoyang syndrome, with poor appetite, anger, irregular menstruation and fluctuation of chills and fever due to the dominance of the liver over the spleen; the blackish blue cheeks of patients with vertigo and vomiting are due to headache caused by reversal of phlegm; the pale blue facial color in young babies with night crying, cold hands and feet, no desire to suck milk and bent back is due to attack of cold pathogens in the spleen; a blue facial color may appear in children with acute convulsions due to attack of violent heat pathogens; and in normal subjects fury, fright, fear and attack of cold weather may also produce a blue facial color.

(3) *Yellow color:*

The yellow facial color usually appears in deficient patients and in patients with diseases of the spleen and stomach or diseases caused by dampness pathogens. Light yellow is a normal facial color of the yellow race, like the people of China, Japan, Korea, Mongolia, Vietnam, Thailand and Singapore.

A pale yellow and sallow facial color is due to injury of the spleen and stomach; a yellow facial color in obese patients is due to accumulation of phlegm and dampness pathogens in the stomach; a yellow facial color in wasted patients is due to fire pathogens in the stomach; a yellow color in the eyes and skin of the whole body is a physical sign of jaundice; a fresh yellow facial color is due to attack by cold and dampness pathogens; a yellow facial color with edema is due to accumulation of dampness in a deficient spleen; a sallow complexion is due to deficiency and weakness of the heart and spleen or malnutrition; a yellow facial color in chronic patients with unimpaired appetite is due to attack by endogerous heat pathogens; a yellow facial color in withered patients is due to attack of deficient heat pathogens to the stomach; a yellow and dry face is due to depletion of body fluid caused by heat pathogens; a dull yellow facial color is due to exhaustion of body fluid; a light yellow facial color is due to the attack of cold pathogens to a deficient stomach; and a mixed facial color of yellow and white is due to the attack of cold pathogens to a deficient spleen and stomach.

A yellow face, cornea and skin all over the body is a physical sign of jaundice. The yellow color of jaundice may be either bright or dull. The fresh yellow color like orange peel appears in patients with Yang jaundice due to attack of damp-heat pathogens; and the dull smoky yellow color in patients of Yin jaundice is due to attack of cold and dampness pathogens. Jaundice may appear in patients with acute icteric hepatitis, cholecystitis, liver cirrhosis, chronic hepatitis and liver cancer.

A dark yellow color of the face with red spots and blood streaks may appear in liver cirrhosis with ascites patients; a yellow facial color with pale lips may appear in diarrhea patients; a yellow color on the bulb of the nose in obese patients is due to accumulation of cold pathogens in the chest; a bluish yellow color on the bulb of the nose may appear in patients with stranguria; a yellow facial color with edema may appear in chronic wasted patients with poor appetite and weakness of the body; an overwhelming yellow facial color may appear in chronic patients; a light yellow facial color in patients with repeated sighing, running nose with clear discharge, chills or fever is due to common cold caused by wind-cold pathogens; a golden yellow color of the skin of a newborn baby is called fetal jaundice; the appearance of an apparent yellow color on the bulb of the nose, forehead and whole face indicates the alleviation of disease; a yellow color appearing on the tip and bridge of the nose and canthi of the eyes indicates the improvement of disease; and a yellow color and edema of face, bluish yellow color or alternate color between yellow and white may appear in children with indigestive malnutrition with ascites and engorgement of the veins of the abdominal wall.

(4) *White color:*

A white facial color is related to diseases of the lungs and colon, diseases caused by cold pathogens or diseases in deficient patients with depletion of blood or qi. The white color is produced by coagulation of blood in meridians caused by cold pathogens or due to deficiency of qi and blood or depletion of qi and blood in meridians.

A white facial color with a red tint and bright piercing eyes are the normal facial appearance of healthy subjects; a pale complexion may appear in patients with severe abdominal pain due to attack of endogenous cold pathogens or chills due to attack of external cold pathogens; a snow-white and puffy face indicates deficiency of Yang qi; a light white facial color may appear in patients with deficiency of Ying (nutrient) and blood; a sudden pale complexion or white facial color without luster may appear in patients with profuse cold sweating due to sudden loss of Yang qi (vital energy); a light white facial color in patients with abdominal distension, increase of intestinal gurgling sound, diarrhea, bent back and cold limbs is due to accumulation of cold pathogens in the body; coughing in patients with snow-white facial color, profuse clear thin sputum and running nose with clear discharge is caused by cold pathogens; a white emaciated face with red cheeks and lips, hot sensation in the heart, palms and soles, night sweating and insomnia is due to deficiency of Yin and excessiveness of fire pathogens; a bloodless complexion with white nose bulb is due to loss of blood and deficiency of blood; a snow-white facial color may appear in patients of cold syndrome with body rolled up and covered with a thick blanket; a bluish white facial color may occur in patients of cold syndrome with cold tip of the nose and cool exhaled air; white spots or patches may appear on the face of patients with intestinal parasites; depigmented patches may appear on the face of patients of vitiligo without any discomfort.

White patches may appear on the faces of patients with the following skin diseases:

1) Simple pityriasis in children and young people.

2) Tinea vesicolor on the face, front chest and back of young people. This is an infectious skin disease with lesions scattered on the face, neck and trunk, but the skin lesions on the face may often be misdiagnosed. The color of the lesions may change with the season — white in summer and yellow or dark brown in winter.

3) Vitiligo: The early skin lesions are porcelain-white spots in a size from a pinpoint to a soybean, and then they may increase in size to form round patches or stripes and spread to almost the whole face, with the eyebrows, eyelashes and beard turning white.

4) Solar white patches: These are skin lesions caused by exposure to sunlight and common in aged people, without any bad effect on the body. They may gradually disappear.

A pale complexion and palpitations of the heart may be caused by fear; the quick exchange of white and red facial color in patients with floating and rapid pulse may be due to shame. These are not pathological facial colors. A white, dry and thin face is due to exhaustion of blood. Liver diseases in patients with white facial color are difficult to treat.

(5) *Black color:*

The black facial color is related to diseases of the kidneys and urinary bladder, and diseases with pain or caused by deficiency of the kidneys or cold pathogens. The black color is produced by accumulation of cold pathogens, stagnation of qi and blood or deficiency of kidney Yin or Yang.

A dark black facial color may appear in chronic patients with deficiency of kidney essence or stasis of blood; a bluish black facial color is due to severe pain, blood stasis or accumulation of cold pathogens; a dull black facial color is due to deficiency of kidney Yang and impaired metabolism of body fluid; a greyish black skin over the orbital region is due to deficiency of the kidneys, accumulation of body fluid or attack of cold and dampness pathogens; a light black color on the nose bulb is due to accumulation of water in the body; a smoky color underneath the eyes is due to accumulation of phlegm and body fluid; a dark black facial color may appear in patients of Xiaxiao (lower type of diabetes mellitus) with thin body, dry ears and turbid urine as an oily liquid; and dry nostrils with smoky black color are due to attack of violent toxic heat pathogens.

In normal persons, a bluish black color underneath the eyes and dusty complexion may be the prodromal signs of sickness; blue or black canthi of the eyes indicate the onset of a critical disease; a foggy and smoky complexion indicates a lingering disease; and a dry and roasted complexion indicates injury to the internal organs by heat and fire pathogens and exhaustion of kidney essence.

As mentioned in an ancient medical book entitled *Diagnosis Along Meridians*: "The sudden appearance of edema in patients with a black face is a sign of death; sufferers from true heart pain with black face and cold extremities may die within one day; and the disease of a patient with a bluish black facial color, small staring eyes and oily sweating is difficult to treat because of the invasion of pathogens into the solid organs."

III. Pathological Facial Features and Diagnosis of Diseases

The normal face should look vigorous and vivid, and at the same time it should not show distress, mental or spiritual disturbance, anemia, jaundice or edema. These are the normal facial features; but how about the pathological facial features?

(1) *Facial features and diagnosis of diseases:*
1) Obese or thin face: Corpulent people with obese faces are full of dampness pathogens and phlegm in the body; and the lean people with thin faces are full of fire pathogens and susceptible to coughing. Obese people hate physical exertion, and tend to spend a lot of time lying down and sleeping. They often suffer from symptoms of deficiency of Yang qi and accumulation of phlegm and dampness pathogens, and they are susceptible to stroke (apoplexy). Thin people like physical activity and mental work, and they often suffer from chronic cough and symptoms of deficiency of Yin and blood or excessiveness of ministerial fire. The are fond of physical activities, good at meditation and susceptible to worries.

2) Edema of the face: This edema usually appear on the parts of face with much loose connective tissue. The thickness of the upper eyelid is a criterion for diagnosis of edema, and an apparently thickened upper eyelid is reliable evidence of edema. The forehead and the area between the eyebrows with thin skin and flat bone surface are ideal places for detecting pitting edema. Facial edema may appear in both general and local diseases.

3) Deviation of the mouth and eyes: This symptom may appear in patients with facial palsy or hemiplegia after a cerebrovascular accident.

4) Swelling and pain in the cheeks with fever: This is a symptom of mumps (epidemic parotitis) in children.

5) Unsymmetrical face: The hypertrophy or atrophy of one

25

side of the face may occur in patients with wryneck, congenital unilateral hypertrophy of the face, unilateral atrophy of the face, brain injury or encephalitis.

(2) *Pathological facial features and diagnosis of diseases:*
1) Acute diseases: Flushed face, restlessness, fluttering alae of the nose, blisters on the lips and distressing facial expression may appear in patients of acute febrile diseases, such as lobar pneumonia and malaria.

2) Chronic diseases: Withered face with a dark gray or pale color and dull eyes may appear in patients with chronic wasting diseases, such as cancer, cirrhosis of the liver and tuberculosis.

3) Rheumatic heart disease: A sallow and puffy face with purplish red cheeks, cynotic lips and mixed colors of yellow, red and purple (or blue), palpitations of the heart and dyspnea may occur in patients of rheumatic heart disease.

4) Anemia: Pale face, lips and tongue, tired expression and weakness of the body may appear in various anemic patients.

5) Mucoid edema: A broad, pale and edematous face with dull eyes, sluggish response, sparse hair and eyebrows, and pale and puffy tongue may appear in patients with hypothyroidism.

6) Hyperthyroidism: Alarming facial expression, increased eye fissure, protruding eyeballs, twinkling eyes, high excitability, annoyance and anger may appear in patients with hyperthyroidism.

7) Acromegaly: Enlarged skull, elongated face, forward protruding chin, bulging superciliary arches and zygomatic bones, thickened lips and tongue, and large nose and ears may appear in patients of acromegaly.

8) Wry-smiling face: Locked jaw, and spasm of the facial

26

muscles with a wry smile may appear in patients of tetanus.

9) Severe dehydration: Withered face with bulging zygomatic bones and sharpened nose bridge, dry lips and tongue, greyish white face, apathetic eyes and cool sweat on the forehead may appear in patients with dehydration caused by severe vomiting and diarrhea.

10) Liver diseases: The face is bluish grey or yellowish blue in color, dull, lusterless, puffy, dry and withered, with bluish grey skin around the orbits and canthi of the eyes in patients of liver diseases with high irritability, anger and indigestion.

11) Typhoid fever: Apathetic face and retarded response may appear in patients of intestinal typhoid fever, cerebrospinal meningitis or encephalitis with high fever.

12) Moon-shaped face: Moon-shaped or balloon-like face with a color as dark as a red date with many acne-type skin lesions and enlarged hair follicle pores may appear in patients with hypersecretion of the adrenal cortical hormones.

13) Mask face: Apathetic and dull face like a mask due to relaxation of the facial mimetic muscles may appear in patients of Parkinson's disease.

14) High fever: Flushed face, quick breath and fluttering alae of the nose may appear in patients with high fever.

15) Muscular atrophy: Depressed cheeks, loose lips, drooping of the lower lip, ptosis of the upper eyelids and having difficulty in opening the eyes may appear in patients with muscular atrophy.

16) Cretinism: Underdeveloped childish face with dull expression, broad and flat nose bridge, widely separated eyes, swollen eyelids, narrow eye fissures, rough skin, dry and sparse hair, low forehead, upward tilted nose and large and thick tongue often protruding from the mouth may appear in children

suffering from cretinism, a congenital disease due to hypofunction of the thyroid gland in the infant stage.

17) Hypo-ovarianism: The apparent vegetations below the inner canthi, big ears, small chin, webbed neck, low posterior hair border, cubitus valgus and short body height may appear in patients with hypo-ovarianism, a congenital disease due to sex chromosome abnormality.

18) Pulmonary tuberculosis: Emaciated and snow-white face with bright red cheeks in the afternoon, glittering eyes, tidal fever, night sweating, cough and poor appetite may appear in patients of pulmonary tuberculosis.

19) Measles: Besides fever, cough and sneezing, slightly congested eyes, photophobia, weeping, increase of discharge from the eyes and running nose are the prodromal symptoms before appearance of skin rashes in patients of measles.

20) Cyanosis: Cyanotic lips and cheeks due to anoxia and increase of reduced hemoglobin in the blood may appear in children with congenital heart diseases and in adults above middle age with heart diseases or chronic respiratory diseases.

21) Acne rosacea (brandy nose): Oily and flushed face, more remarkable in the central area of the face, including the tip of the nose, alae of the nose and cheeks may appear in adults with early lesions of diffuse telangeictatic erythema with scattered small papules, nodules and pustules, and late lesion of hypertrophic tuberculate rhinophyma (hammer-nose).

22) Epidemic hemorrhagic fever: Flushed face like that of a drunken person, with red neck and upper chest, yellow scelera, headache, lumbago, pain of the whole body and fever may appear in patients of epidemic hemorrhagic fever.

23) CO poisoning: Cherry-red face, lips and conjunctiva of the eyes, dizziness, weakness, palpitations of the heart,

vomiting, mental confusion, coma and even death may appear in severe cases of CO poisoning.

24) Cancers: Pale and withered face, and emaciated body are common physical signs of patients with cancer.

25) Hepatolenticular degeneration: Dull and fixed eyes, watering in the mouth, slurred speech or aphasia may appear in patients of hepatolenticular degeneration, a familial cirrhosis of the liver and neurological disease with psychotic symptoms, such as unreasonable crying and laughing.

26) Scarlet fever: Flushed face, pale color around the mouth, strawberry tongue and fever are the specific physical signs and symptoms of scarlet fever.

27) Epidemic parotitis (mumps): Big mouth, swelling around the ear lobe without a clear margin, and red color, hotness, swelling and tenderness over the parotid glands may appear in children suffered from epidemic parotitis, a viral epidemic disease occurring in spring and autumn.

28) Congenital heart diseases: Cyanotic lips may appear in children, more remarkable during crying and struggling, with a tendency to squat down after violent exercise.

29) Ascariasis: Sallow face with red lips and small milia like fine pieces of broken rice scattered over the forehead and cheekbones without pain or itching may appear in children with ascaris.

30) Melanosis: Punctate pigmentation in pale or dark brown or dark grey color may fuse together to form large patches without clear boundaries, and they may appear on the forehead and cheekbones or around the orbital regions of patients with melanosis caused by long-term contact with tar, lead, arsenic or mercury.

31) Scleroderma: Hard facial skin without wrinkles, apa-

thetic face, pointed nose, small mouth difficult to completely close, hard skin on the trunk and limbs, and inflexible fingers with limitation of movement may appear in patients with scleroderma, a chronic skin disease with cause unknown.

32) Left heart failure: Pale and edematous face, distressed expression, sweating, severe cough with pink foamy sputum and dyspnea may appear in patients with congestive failure of the left side of the heart.

33) Eunuchism (absence of testis): Pale face without beard, delicate facial skin with many wrinkles and thick folds of skin in clumps on the peripheral area of the face and neck may appear in patients of eunuchism.

34) Diabetes mellitus: Yellowish white face with red papules, faded away under pressure and the telangiectatic erythema patches with smooth surface, yellow depressed central area and red peripheral zone may appear in patients of diabetes mellitus.

35) Pale complexion: A pale complexion may appear in patients with malnutrition, anemia, edema, chronic wasting diseases, forced indoor life deprived of sunlight and ultraviolet light for a long time, severe abdominal pain, chills, acute blood hemorrhage, shock, overfatigue and violent mental stress.

36) Dark complexion: A brownish black complexion may appear in people who do continuous outdoor work and are constantly exposed to sunshine and wind. A greyish blue facial color may appear in patients with cirrhosis of the liver or in the late stage of liver cancer.

37) White hair and ruddy complexion: A ruddy face due to hemorrhage of superficial capillary blood vessels may appear in aged patients with arteriosclerosis.

38) Physiological cyanosis at high altitudes: Cyanosis of the lips, tongue, ear auricle, cheek, fingers and toes (more remark-

able in the lips, conjunctiva of eyes and finger) often occur in people first visiting high altitudes, with a severity of cyanosis in proportion to the altitude, which may spontaneously disappear 3-4 weeks later.

39) Critical complexion: Pale or lead grey and withered face, apathetic expression, spiritless eyes, depressed orbits and sharp nose bone may appear in patients with profuse hemorrhage, severe shock, dehydration or acute peritonitis.

In brief, the observation of facial color and expression is very useful in the diagnosis of diseases. The normal facial color of yellow race is light yellow with a red tinge.

In addition, patients with jaundice, leukemia and pigmentation may also show marked change of facial color.

IV. Inspection of Face and Diagnosis of Diseases

1. The three divisions of the face:

As shown in Fig. 2-1, the part of the face above the eyebrows is called the upper third of the face, and is related to diseases of the brain; the part between the eyebrows and the lower border of the nose is called the middle third of the face, and is related to diseases of the respiratory system; and the part below the nose is called the lower third of the face, and related to diseases of the digestive system.

2. Important points for attention in inspection of the face:

1) A symmetrical face is an important feature of normal subjects.

2) Blue color around the outer canthus is an indication of diseases of the uterus in women.

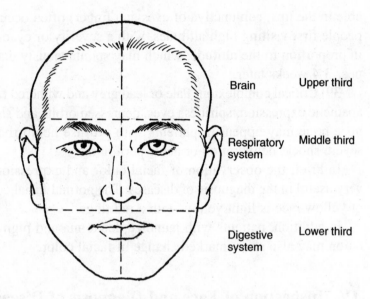

Fig. 2-1 Basic diagram of facial features

3) Heavy eyebrows, large round nose, thick lips and short thick neck are typical features of healthy men full of vigor.

4) People with medially deviated eyeballs or uneven sizes of eyeballs are susceptible to cerebral hemorrhage; and subjects with laterally deviated eyeballs are susceptible to cancer.

3. Relation of facial color to health:

1) Gloomy color: A gloomy mixed color of blue, white and purple may appear in patients with deterioration of disease or in people with unstable mental condition.

2) Dark color: This color is darker than the gloomy color but with a similar significance; and a purplish black color on the forehead also indicates deterioration of disease.

3) Dark red color: This indicates deep anger.

4) Purplish black color: This indicates anoxia and excessive carbon dioxide in the blood.

5) Pink color: This is a healthy facial color of normal subjects.

4. Inspection of forehead and diagnosis of diseases:

1) A bright forehead indicates good health; a black forehead indicates a serious sickness.

2) Black color on the upper part of the forehead indicates a critical prognosis of disease, because the color of the forehead can show the change of the frontal lobe of the brain. An abnormal color may appear on the upper part of the forehead in patients with accumulation of feces in the transverse colon. A bright forehead indicates the amelioration of disease; and dirty spots may appear on the forehead in pregnant women or patients with pulmonary tuberculosis or diseases of the uterus.

3) Blue engorged veins in the shape of earthworms may appear in the areas of the face lateral to both eyes in people susceptible to apoplexy (stroke); engorged veins on the left temporal region indicate the accumulation of feces in the sigmoid colon; appearing on the right temporal region, they indicate accumulation of feces in the cecum. The accumulation of feces may cause numbness of the contralateral hand and foot.

4) The upper part of the forehead is closely related to the kidneys, and a plump forehead indicates normal kidney function; gloomy color and dirty spots below the anterior hairline indicate diseases of the kidneys.

5. Inspection of the glabella (area between eyebrows) and diagnosis of diseases:

1) Children with engorged blue veins in this area are sus-

ceptible to common cold and diseases of the nervous and digestive systems. This also indicates the accumulation of feces in a new-born baby.

2) White color in this area indicates severe mental fatigue.

3) A vertical wrinkle in this area may appear in people susceptible to hypertension or heart disease.

4) Wrinkles in this area may appear in people susceptible to neurasthenia and indigestion.

6. Inspection of the lower jaw and diagnosis of diseases:

1) A purplish black color on the lower jaw indicates disease in the lower abdomen.

2) Patients with forward protruded chin may have diseases of the tonsils.

7. Inspection of the cheeks and diagnosis of diseases:

1) The cheeks are closely related to the lungs. If the skin and muscles of the cheeks are soft and plump, and the color of the cheeks is yellow with a red tint, the function of the lungs should be good. Flushed cheeks indicate poor lung function.

2) Sharp cheeks with less muscle and fat tissue indicates deficiency and weakness of the lungs, and flushed sharp cheeks indicate susceptibility to pneumonia.

3) The appearance of a red spider-like capillary network on the cheeks indicates alcoholic cirrhosis of the liver.

4) People with plump cheeks usually have strong stomachs and impaired kidney function; but people with depressed cheeks may have a weak stomachs but good kidney function.

V. Inspection of Facial Patterns and Diagnosis of Diseases

1. Different facial patterns (Fig.2-2):

1) Tuberculosis type: Long and narrow face, and short distance between the eyes.

2) Kidney type: Long and narrow face, and wide distance between the eyes.

3) Peptic ulcer type: A facial pattern between the above two types, with depressed eyeballs and the average distance between the eyes neither too short nor very wide.

4) Pernicious anemia type: A wide face, especially wide lower jaw and the wide distance between the eyes.

5) Gallbladder type: Round wide face and narrow distance between the eyes.

2. Inspection of facial pattern and diagnosis of diseases:

1) Tuberculosis type: Faces of this type are long and narrow, with a sharp chin and short distance between the eyes. People with this kind of face are susceptible to infection of tuberculous bacilli. People of this type with a respiratory body constitution are more susceptible to pulmonary tuberculosis.

2) Kidney type: Faces of this type are long and narrow, with a wide distance between the eyes. People with this type of face are susceptible to bacterial infection of the kidneys. Kidney diseases are often complicated with hypertension.

3) Peptic ulcer (internal organ ptosis) type: People of this type have a facial pattern intermediate between the above two types, average distance between eyes and depressed eyeballs. They are susceptible to peptic ulcer of the stomach. Their neck

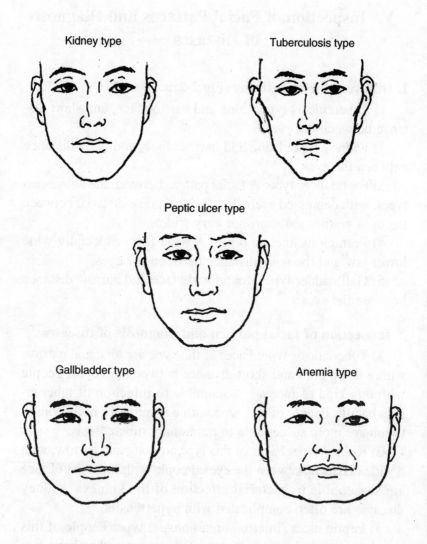

Fig.2-2　Facial patterns and susceptible diseases

is shorter than that of the tuberculosis type.

4) Pernicious anemia type: In patients of this type, the whole face is large and wide, the lower part of the face is wider, the lower jaw makes a sharp angle, the distance between eyes is very wide, the distance between the lower end of the nose and the border of the upper lip is short, the facial color is bluish or pale, and bruises may appear on the skin over prominent parts of the body.

5) Gallbladder type: People of this type usually have a wide round face, and round lower jaw, narrower than that of the anemia type, and their face is red in color or red with a blackish purple tint. They are susceptible to gallstones. A pale complexion indicates diseases of the kidneys. People of respiratory, muscular and mixed type of body constitution are also susceptible to gallstones.

Chapter 3
INSPECTION OF THE EYES, EARS AND NOSE, AND DIAGNOSIS OF DISEASES

The eyes are the display windows of the mind, showing the changes of emotions and the state of health of the human body. The eyes are thus a thermometer of the health of human body.

The ears are the hearing organs, which perceive sound. As mentioned in the *Miraculous Pivot*, an ancient medical book: "Kidney qi is supplied to the ears. The ears can hear different sounds only if the kidneys are normal." The ears are gathering places of vessels and external orifices of the heart; the liver and gallbladder meridians pass through the ears; the binding acupoint of the lung meridian is in the ears; and all the orifices of the sense organs may be blocked if the spleen function is impaired. Therefore, pathological changes of the above organs may be shown on their correspondent projecting areas on the ears.

The nose is an external orifice of the lungs, and the breath passes through it. Besides respiration, it is also in charge of smelling and phonation. The meridians of the lungs, kidneys, spleen, stomach and gallbladder are all connected with the nose. Therefore, inspection of the nose can be applied to diagnose diseases of the whole body.

In brief, the eyes, ears and nose are important sense organs on the face, and at the same time they can be used to diagnose general diseases as well as to show the state of health of the human body.

I. Inspection of the Eyes and Diagnosis of Diseases

1. Diagnosis of eye diseases:

1) Hordeolum (stye): This is a small hard nodule on the eyelid with local redness and swelling, and a yellow pustule may be formed a few days later. Premature incision and squeezing of the pustule is dangerous, because it may threaten life. Patients with repeated relapses of stye should be carefully examined, to rule out diabetes mellitus.

2) Entropion of the eyelid and trichiasis: Trichiasis may occur independently or as a complication of entropion of the eyelid with the symptoms of conjunctival congestion, photophobia and shedding tears.

3) Fetropion of the eyelid: The eyelid may be externally turned up and detached from the eyeball, with exposure of partial or complete balbar conjunctiva, to produce dryness and ulceration of the cornea, shedding tears and impairment of vision.

4) Trachoma: Trachoma is a serious eye disease leading to blindness, and the patients may suffer from congestion, turbidity and thickening of the conjunctiva, with opaque blood vessels.

5) Epidemic keroconjunctivitis: This is an epidemic eye disease in summer and autumn, with punctate turbid spots on the cornea one week after the onset of the disease, increase of watery discharge from the eyes, follicular proliferation of the

conjunctiva and swollen lymph nodes in front of the ears.

6) Drug-induced conjunctivitis: This is an allergic eye disease, with a burning, pricking and itching sensation in the eyes, conjunctival congestion, edema and increased serious excretion of the eyes; severe cases may include eczema and exudate on the eyelids.

7) Spring conjunctivitis: This is an allergic eye disease in children common in spring, with intractable itching in the eyes, conjunctival congestion, photophobia, and shedding tears with sticky secretion. It may be spontaneously cured.

8) Pterygium: This is the proliferative tissue on the balbar conjunctiva in the palpebral fissure caused by chronic stimulation of sunlight and wind in fishermen, farmers and other outdoor workers. The thick pterygium has blood congestion but the thin pterygium has not; and the pterygium can be divided into resting and progressive types. Vision may be interfered with in the late stage.

9) Keratitis: This is a local infection of the cornea, with photophobia, shedding tears, pain, ciliary congestion, corneal turbidity and neoformative blood vessels on the cornea.

10) Cornea softening: This is an eye disease with necrosis, perforation and rupture of the cornea in children, with lingering diarrhea or after-infection of measles, and the children may suffer from night blindness and dryness and dullness of the balbar conjunctiva. It may cause blindness in both eyes.

11) Seleritis: This is a collagen disease of the eye caused by auto-immunity, and is related to tuberculosis, leprosy, syphilis and endocrinal disturbance. The typical physical sign is localized purplish blood congestion on the lesion of the sclera, and iridocyclitis is a complication of this disease.

12) Glaucoma: This is a common dangerous eye disease,

resulting in blindness due to increase of ocular pressure and progressive atrophy of the optic nerve. Patients of open-angle glaucoma may have blurred vision, slight ciliary congestion, slightly dilated pupils, sluggish light reflex and an apparent red and green halo around the light source. Patients of angle-closure glaucoma may have increase of ocular pressure, defect or reduction of the visual field and depression of the optic disc. Glaucoma can be divided into the congenital and secondary types.

13) Cataracts: This is an eye disease with opaque lens. Congenital cataracts in infants is caused by viral infection from German measles, mumps or chicken-pox in pregnant mothers; acquired cataracts in aged people is caused by turbidity in the equatorial cortex of the lens arranged in a radiating pattern. Turbidity of the lens can be clearly observed after the pupil is dilated.

14) Strabismus (squint): This is an eye disease with impairment of contraction of the extra-ocular muscles due to intracranial, intra-orbital or general diseases of the human body, and the patients may show deviation of the eyeball and impairment of movement of the eyeball, and suffer from poor orientation, dizziness and nausea due to double vision.

2. Inspection of the eyes and diagnosis of diseases of the whole body:

(1) *Five wheels of the eyes and diagnosis of diseases:*
According to the theory of the five wheels of the eyes (the blood, wind, qi, water and muscle wheels) in traditional Chinese medicine, the different wheels are correspondingly related to the five internal organs (Fig.3-1).

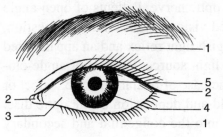

1: muscle wheel (eyelid)—spleen

2: blood wheel (canthi)— heart

3: qi wheel (sclera)—lungs

4: wind wheel (iris)—liver

5: water wheel (pupil)—kidneys

Fig. 3-1

As mentioned in the ancient medical book, *An Exhaustive and Comprehensive Survey of the Silver Sea*: "For inspection of the eyes, the pupils should be observed first, and then the wind wheel, sclera, eyelids and canthi in sequence. The patient should stand straight, with the eyelids slowly opened with the fingers. The pupils are observed first; they may promptly dilate and contract in clear eyes. Then the wind wheel is observed, and the mental activity is normal if the iris can freely dilate and contract. Then the qi wheel is observed, and there is no sickness if the sclera is shiny and smooth. And finally, the muscle wheel is observed, and the eyelids can be forcibly opened and closed in normal subjects, and the canthi are not a dirty red color."

1) Water wheel: The water wheel is the pupil, 2-4 mm in diameter under ordinary light. The brightness of the pupil should be observed first, and then its size and shape. A normal pupil can freely contract and dilate following the change of light — it is smaller in a strong light and larger in a dim light. The pupils should be clean and transparent to clearly observe any

subject. Both pupils should be round in shape and the same size. Excessive dilation or contraction, and change of color and transparency are all abnormal changes in a pupil.

Excessive dilation of a pupil is due to emotional disturbance, loss of essence and qi in the body or upward invasion of phlegm and fire pathogens; dilated pupils may appear in cases of acute diseases, such as apoplexy and in critical patients about to die; the sluggish response or loss of light reflex of pupils may appear in patients with coma; unequal pupils or irregular change of pupil size may be due to diseases of the central nervous system or disturbance of nervous control in the iris; unequal pupils, sluggish or abolished light reflex of pupils and mental confusion may be caused by dysfunction of the midbrain; and the bilateral dilation of pupils and loss of light reflex are physical signs of dying patients.

Constricted pupils may appear in patients with intoxication of chloropromazine, barbitals, morphine, organic phosphorous compounds and chloral hydrate, and the constriction is in proportion to the severity of intoxication; this condition may also occur in patients with epidemic encephalitis B and paralysis of the sympathetic nerves. The pupils of aged people are smaller than those of young people, because of deficiency of kidney qi. The reduction of the pupils in size is usually caused by injury to the liver and kidneys, or deficiency of vital energy.

2) Wind wheel (iris): The wind wheel is related to the liver, because the wind in the body is controlled by the liver. The upward protrusion of the upper border of the iris to form a dome is due to stagnation of excessive liver qi in meridians, poor dispersion of liver qi and upward accumulation of excessive qi.

A purplish red halo in a deep layer around the iris and arranged in a radiating pattern is due to blood stasis caused by excessive fire pathogens in the liver and gallbladder.

The vision may be interfered with by a layer of greyish white turbid membrane in the deep layer over the iris, produced by toxic heat pathogens in the liver and gallbladder, which can attack the eyes, consume body fluid and cause stasis and co-agulation of blood.

In children with indigestive malnutrition, complication of the eyes is a serious disease with turbid fluid in the anterior chamber, and ulcerated and softened cornea of the eyes.

3) Qi wheel (sclera): The qi wheel is related to the lungs, because qi in the body is controlled by the lungs.

The yellow color on the sclera of jaundice is an early physi-cal sign of liver disease: Red sclera indicates diseases of the heart; white sclera indicates diseases of the lungs; blue sclera indicates diseases of the liver and black sclera indicates dis-eases of the kidneys. In patients with red eye disease (acute conjunctivitis), the sclera is fresh red in color, with a hot sensation, shedding tears and difficulty in opening the eyes, and it is an infectious eye disease caused by toxic wind-heat patho-gens and transmitted by the dirty secretion of the eyes. The bluish grey or purplish blue spots on the sclera are produced by attack of toxic heat and fire pathogens. Red nodules like immovable red beans protruding from the sclera without defi-nite location are caused by toxic fire pathogens accumulated in the lungs, stagnation of wind, dampness and heat pathogens in the eye collaterals, and may also be caused by some general diseases of the body. The pterygium on the sclera may cover the cornea or protrude from the palpebral fissure, and it is caused by stagnation of toxic heat pathogens in the spleen and stomach produced after eating too much spicy and greasy food.

4) Blood wheel (canthi of eye): The blood wheel is related

to the heart, because the blood is controlled by the heart.

In normal canthi of the eye, the fine blood vessels are red and vivid in appearance, without sticky and turbid discharge, and no blood vessels spread onto the cornea. The lacrimal gland and duct are patent.

The fine branches of the blood vessels spread from the canthus through the sclera onto the cornea are caused by accumulated heat pathogens in Sanjiao (triple energizer), flaming up of heart fire, wasting of essence and blood, and upward attack of deficient fire due to anxiety or sexual intemperance. Lacrimation from the canthi of the eyes induced by attack of wind is caused by deficiency of liver blood, deficiency of qi and blood, invasion of wind pathogens and loss of control of lacrimation. The continuous shedding of tears is due to extreme sadness or deficiency of liver and kidney Yin, disturbance of the metabolism of the body fluids, upward flaming of deficient fire and loss of control of lacrimation. Red inner canthus is produced by upward flaming of heart fire; and red outer canthus is caused by accumulation of fire in the gallbladder. Red canthi, shedding tears, red cheeks as shown in a drunken person, with cold fingers, are the prodromal symptoms of measles, and the canthi of the eyes are red in patients of typhoid fever.

5) Muscle wheel (eyelid): The muscle wheel is related to the spleen. The normal upper and lower eyelids can freely open and close to protect the eyeballs. The normal eyelid is soft, shiny and yellow in color, the eyelash is regularly arranged along the border of the eyelids and the palpebral conjunctiva is smooth and pink in color.

Dark eyelids indicate deficiency of the kidneys; blue eyelids indicate pain; light red and slightly swollen eyelids and a tired complexion indicate overfatigue; bright eyelids indicate disease caused by accumulation of phlegm and body fluid; dark eyelids indicate diseases caused by cold phlegm; edematous eyelids swollen like balls indicate deficiency of lung and spleen qi or deficiency of spleen and kidney Yang and upward invasion of warm pathogens; ptosis of both upper eyelids, interfering with the vision is due to deficiency of qi and blood, failure of spleen qi to support various organs of body in their normal position, invasion of wind pathogens or congenital deficiency of essence; patients with retracted lower eyelids incapable of covering the eyeballs are susceptible to diseases of the heart and respiratory system; symmetrical edema of both eyelids indicates general diseases of the whole body, such as severe anemia, malnutrition, insomnia, deficiency of the spleen and stomach, menopausal syndrome, chronic liver diseases and angioneurotic edema; unilateral edema of the eyelid is usually caused by local diseases. In normal people, the eyes may twinkle 5-6 times per minute; the eyes may seldom twinkle in patients with insensible cornea, facial palsy or exophthalmic hyperthyroidism; and repeated twinkling of the eyes may appear in patients with irritable conjunctiva, psychological disturbance and hysteria; the failure of closure of the eyes is a symptom of facial palsy; sudden downward staring is a sign of exhaustion of qi and spirit, and indicates a short life span; and automatic twinkling of the eyes may appear in children with dominance of the liver over the spleen caused by an improper diet.

(2) *Inspection of eye color and diagnosis of diseases:*

As mentioned in the *Miraculous Pivot*: "Red color indicates disease of the heart; white indicates disease of the lungs; yellow indicates disease of the spleen; blue indicates disease of

46

the liver; and black indicates disease of the kidneys."

Redness and swelling of the whole eye indicates wind and heat pathogens in the liver; red pupils are due to intra-ocular bleeding; red sclera is due to fire pathogens in the lungs; red eyelids with erosion is due to fire pathogens in the spleen; swelling and redness of the upper eyelids is due to wind-heat pathogens in the spleen; and swelling and redness of the lower eyelids is due to fire and heat pathogens in the stomach; redness in the canthi of the eye is due to fire pathogens in the heart; redness and erosion of the inner canthus is due to invasion of wind-heat pathogens to Shangjiao (upper energizer); redness and erosion of the outer canthus is due to accumulation of heat pathogens in the gallbladder; pale red color in the sclera is due to deficient heat pathogens; and red eyes, red face, tremor of the head, locked jaw, opisthotonus and stiffness of the neck and back are the physical signs of tetanus.

Black eyes in patients with moaning and difficulty in walking is due to invasion of cold and dampness pathogens into the bones; greyish black color below the eyes is due to accumulation of cold rheum in the body; dim color in the eyelids is due to deficiency of the kidneys; bright color in the eyelids is due to retention of rheum; black eyelids, ashen face and flaccid limbs are due to retention of wind phlegm in the body; a blue or dark grey halo around the eyes is due to listlessness, tiredness or insomnia; blue color in the canthi is due to liver disease; blue sclera is due to invasion of liver wind to the lungs; black eyes and pale face are due to emptying of blood vessels and loss of flushed color; black sclera indicates tuberculosis; bluish purple sclera and hollow and uneven pulse indicates tuberculosis in deficient patients with coagulated blood retained in the body; drunken eyes with tears, hot and flushed cheeks and slightly cold fingers are the prodromal physical signs of poxes and measles; and the reduction of black color in pupils and sluggish light reflex indicate the worsening of eye diseases.

Yellow sclera is due to diseases of the gallbladder; yellow pupil indicates a serious disease; dark yellow color in the sclera indicates indigestive malnutrition; yellow pupils, pale lips and blue spots on a red face are the prodromal physical signs of stroke; a faint color between red and yellow in the eyes of patients with diseases caused by external pathogens indicates the transmission of pathogens from the body's surface to internal organs of the body; yellow eyes and irritation indicate the deterioration of a disease; light yellow eyes indicate diarrhea due to deficiency of the spleen; and yellow sclera indicates retardation of urination. Yellow is a normal eye color in aged people.

White pupil is due to cataracts or turbidity of the cornea; white eyes and red face are due to anxiety; pale white canthus is due to deficiency of blood; white eyes and black face are due to wasting of kidney qi; pale white or light yellow pupils indicate deficiency of the kidneys; pale conjunctiva indicates anemia; pale and slightly puffy eyelids, shortness of breath, palpitations of the heart, low speaking voice, spontaneous sweating and general weakness are due to deficient cold pathogens in the spleen and stomach, and deficiency of qi and blood; black eyelids may appear in patients with allergic rhinitis and sinusitis; and greyish black eyelids may appear in women with leukorrhagia, amenorrhea and dysmenorrhea.

(3) *Inspection of the movement of the eyeballs and diagnosis of diseases:*

The normal eyeball is like a ball or pearl, and it can freely turn around. A protruded, depressed or deviated eyeball is an abnormal physical sign.

Protruded eyeball usually appears in patients with hyperthyroidism or intraorbital tumor; depressed eyeball may appear in patients with local inflammation; deviation of the eyeball to different degrees and in various directions is due to deficiency of qi and blood in internal organs or relaxation of muscles and dilation of blood vessels caused by invasion of wind pathogens into a deficient body.

The sudden deviation and limitation of eyeball movement with double vision is due to deficiency of the spleen and blockage of collaterals by phlegm and wind pathogens; sudden protrusion of a red eyeball from the palpebral fissure is due to accumulation of wind and heat pathogens in the five internal solid organs, prompt increase of Yang pathogens and upward attack of toxic heat pathogens, blocking orifices; downward inclination of the eyeball, like the sinking sun at sunset and limitation of movement of the eyeball is due to attack of wind and cold pathogens to the extra-ocular muscles and optic nerve; upward deviation of a single eyeball is due to deficiency of vital energy, weakness of subcutaneous interstices (defensive structures) and invasion of external pathogens, or is caused by external injury; and upward deviation of both eyeballs is due to disturbance of mental activity by upward attack of excessive fire and heat pathogens.

(4) *Inspection of eyelash and tears, and diagnosis of diseases:*

In a healthy person black and sleek eyelashes are regularly arranged. The loss of eyelash reflex is a bad sign of a critical ailment; crying without tears is normal in babies below two months; the absence of tears in older children and adults is due to disturbance of secretion of the lacrimal gland; the absence of tears is due to deficiency of liver and kidney Yin, deficiency of Yin and blood, and exhaustion of body fluid in febrile diseases; itching and dryness in the eyes without tears is due to insufficiency of blood and attack of wind pathogens; shedding of tears with itching and swollen eyelids is due to insufficiency of qi and blood; constant shedding of cool tears with poor vision is due to deficiency of liver and kidney Yin; shedding of hot tears may appear in patients with heat syndrome; and shedding of tears due to cough and asthma may appear in patients with severe cough caused by wind-cold pathogens or whooping cough.

The constant shedding of tears may appear in patients with eyelids incapable of normal opening and closing, or blockage and constriction of the lacrimal duct due to rhinitis, external trauma, nasal polyps, deviation of the nasal septum or tumor in the nose; poor contraction of the orbicular muscle or scar formation on the lacrimal sac may also cause poor drainage of tears; and inflammation of the lacrimal duct, as in patients with styes, may also cause constant shedding of tears.

(5) *Inspection of the brightness of eyes and diagnosis of diseases:*
Normal eyes with good vision should show a clear and bright appearance, with a clear-cut margin between the black iris and white sclera.

A face like a dull mask with spiritless staring eyes is a facial appearance of psychiatric patients; eyes with dirty sclera, dark cornea, blurred vision, but without tears or gum are considered to be spiritless eyes; vertigo and blurred vision is due to deficiency of liver and kidney qi; and lusterless eyes with blurred vision is due to deficiency of blood and body fluid.

(6) *Inspection of the eyebrows and diagnosis of diseases:*

In general, the eyebrows of children are narrow, sparse and pale; they are thick and dense in youths; and the tips of the eyebrows are much longer in aged people. The eyebrows of male youths are broad, dense, dark and long, while they are narrow, long, curved and pale in women. This is a normal variation of eyebrows in human beings.

Sparse eyebrows may appear in patients with endocrinal dysfunction due to necrosis, tumor, inflammation or incision of the pituitary gland; sparse eyebrows are a prodromal sign of mucoid edema and leprosy; complete loss of eyebrows may appear in patients with leprosy, presenility, alopecia areata and alopecia totalis; and white eyebrows may appear in patients with vitiligo and viral iridocyclitis.

(7) *Inspection of the eyes and diagnosis of general diseases:*

The eyes are closely related to the organs in the body, and the early symptoms of some diseases may first appear in the eyes. The common diseases with symptoms appearing in the eyes are as follows:

1) Severe anemia: Retinal bleeding and pale fundus of the eye may appear in patients with severe anemia.

2) Polycythemia: Retinal bleeding, purplish red, engorged and tortional veins on the retina and dark red retina may appear in patients with polycythemia.

3) Leukemia: Pale fundus, retinal bleeding and engorged and tortional veins may appear in patients with leukemia. The local infiltration or nodules may appear on the eyelids or mass in the orbit of one or both eyes, causing protrusion of the eye.

It is called chloroma and more common in children with acute or subacute granulocytic leukemia.

4) Acute nephritis: Edema of the eyelids may appear in patients with acute nephritis.

5) Diabetes mellitus: Thickness of the lens is increased, producing a transient myopia within a short period when the blood sugar is increased; transient hyperopia may occur when the blood sugar is decreased; and the vision is normal when the disease is under control.

6) Chronic nephritis and uremia: Constriction and reduction of the calibor or retinal artery, retinal edema and flocculent exudate may appear in patients with chronic nephritis with uremia; and edema of the optic disc may appear in severe cases.

7) Gout: Superficial scleritis and uveitis may appear in patients with gout.

8) Deficiency of vitamin A: Night blindness and dryness of the cornea and conjunctiva may appear in patients with this disease.

9) Deficiency of vitamin B_1: Retrobulbar neuritis may appear in people drinking too much alcohol over a long period of time or in breast-feeding women.

10) Deficiency of vitamin B_2: Keratitis and neoformation of corneal blood vessels may appear in patients with this disease.

11) Deficiency of vitamin C: Subcutaneous bleeding of the eyelids, subconjunctival bleeding and retinal bleeding may appear in patients with this disease, and intra-orbital bleeding with protrusion of the eyeballs may appear in children.

12) Rheumatic fever and rhematoid arthritis: Kuperficial keratitis, keratitis and iridocyclitis may appear in patients with these diseases.

13) Influenza: Conjunctivitis and optic neuritis may appear in patients with influenza.

14) Infectious hepatitis: Icteric sclera and tiredness of the eyes may appear in patients with hepatitis, and night blindness may occur in severe cases.

15) Scarlet fever with septicemia: Metastatic internal ophthalmitis, and orbital cellulitis may appear in patients with this disease.

16) Tuberculosis: Vesicular keratoconjunctivitis, scleritis, choroiditis, retinal periphlebitis and optic neuritis may appear in patients with tuberculosis.

17) Ascariasis: Edema and urticaria on the eyelids may occur in patients with ascaris.

18) Malaria: Keratitis caused by herpes simplex virus may appear in patients with malaria with high fever.

19) Cerebral schitosomiasis: Septic edema and secondary optic nerve atrophy may appear in patients with this disease.

20) Measles: Conjunctivitis may appear in the early stage, and cornea softening in the late stage of this disease.

21) Chickenpox: Vesicles may appear on the eyelids, conjunctiva and cornea in patients with chickenpox.

22) Epidemic parotitis (mumps): Iridocyclitis and keratitis may occur in patients with this disease.

23) Epidemic encephalitis B: Paralysis of the extra-ocular muscles, failure of accommodation and dilation or spastic constriction of the pupils, sluggish or abolished light reflex and optic edema during increase of intracranial pressure may appear in patients with this disease, and optic nerve atrophy may appear in the late stage of this disease.

24) Diphtheria: Diphtheric conjunctivitis, keratitis, paralysis of the extra-ocular muscles and failure of accommodation

may appear in patients with diphtheria, but the pupils are normal.

25) Whooping cough: Subcutaneous bleeding of eyelids and subconjunctival bleeding may appear in patients with whooping cough, and retinal bleeding may appear in severe cases.

26) Tuberculous meningitis: Paralysis of the extra-ocular muscles, uneven or dilated pupils, optic neuritis and optic edema may appear in patients with this disease.

27) Hydroencephalus: Optic edema, optic nerve atrophy and downward displacement of the eyeballs with exposure of the upper part of the sclera may occur in patients with hydroencephalus.

28) Electrical injury: Cataracts may appear a few days or a few years after electrical injury, and severe impairment of vision may occur as a result of optic nerve injury.

29) Poisonous snake or insect bite: Kerotoconjunctivitis, dilation of the pupils, impairment of accommodation, ptosis of the eyelids and paralysis of the extra-ocular muscles may appear in patients of poisonous snake or insect bite.

30) Irregular menstruation: Edema of the eyelids, congestion of the conjunctiva, compensatory subconjunctival bleeding, retrobulbar optic neuritis, cyclitis and glaucoma syndrome may appear in women with irregular menstruation.

31) Menopausal syndrome: Headache, tiredness and pain in the eyes right after a short period of reading which can not be relieved by wearing glasses, and dry kerotoconjunctivitis due to reduction of lacrimal excretion may appear in patients with this disease.

32) Migraine: Scintillating dark spots in the central area of the visual field and spreading to its peripheral part with a frequency of more than 10 times per second and lasting for 10-20

minutes may appear before the onset of migraine. Fundoscopic examination of eyes is normal.

33) Neurasthenia: Tiredness of the eyes, poor vision, double vision, photophobia and shedding tears may appear in patients with neurasthenia, but examination finds the eyes to be normal.

34) Hysteria: Sudden blindness in one or both eyes without dilation of the pupils may appear in patients with hysteria. The light reflex is active, the fundoscopic examination is normal and the patients do not dodder as they walk.

35) Rhinitis and sinusitis: Reflective lacrimation may appear in patients with acute rhinitis; congestion, swelling, tenderness and inflammation of the eyelids may appear in patients with acute sinusitis; orbital cellulitis may appear in cases with disseminated inflammation.

36) Tonsilitis: Relaptic iridocyclitis, retinal choroiditis and retrobulbar optic neuritis may appear in patients with tonsilitis.

37) Nasopharyngeal cancer: Paralysis of the extra-ocular muscles and double vision may appear in patients with this tumor, and protrusion of the eyeballs may appear in cases with invasion of tumor into the orbit.

38) Periodontitis and alveolar abscess: Keratitis, sclerotitis, retinitis, optic neuritis and orbital cellulitis may appear in patients with periodontal infection.

39) Herpes simplex: Vesicles may appear on the eyelids, and keratitis caused by herpes simplex virus may occur in patients with this disease.

40) Leprosy: Nodules on the eyelids, loss of eyebrows and eyelashes, small leprotic nodules on the palpebral conjunctiva, sclera, margin of the cornea and surface of the iris, diffuse conjunctivitis, keratitis, scleritis and iridocyclitis may appear in patients with leprosy; incomplete closure of the eyelids in

cases with damage to the facial nerve; dryness of the cornea and conjunctiva due to reduction of lacrimal secretion may occur in cases with damage to the lacrimal glands and paralysis of the extra-ocular muscles and disturbance of movement of the eyes may occur in cases with damage to the abducent and oculomotor nerves.

41) Syphilis: Inflammation of the corneal stroma, syphilitic iridocyclitis and diffuse retinal choroiditis may appear in patients with syphilis; optic neuritis, atrophy of the optic nerve and blindness may occur in cases with damage to the optic nerve.

II. Inspection of the Ears and Diagnosis of Diseases

1. Disturbance of hearing:

(1) *Tinnitus:*

This is a symptom with subjective hearing of a noise in the ears. The noise can be divided into two types: High pitch like the chirping of a cicada is due to deficiency of qi and blood to nourish the ear and deficiency of kidney essence with upward disturbance of deficient fire pathogens; and low pitch is due to upward disturbance of excessive liver and gallbladder fire pathogens or phlegm and turbid dampness pathogens.

(2) *Deafness:*

Deafness in one or both ears may appear in many diseases of the ears, and neurological and medical diseases. Deafness may be divided into the transient and progressive types. In the former type, sudden loss of hearing is usually caused by attack of excessive pathogens, such as wind, heat, dampness and phlegm, blocking the ear orifice; and in the latter type, the gradual reduction and loss of hearing may be caused by deficiency of kidney qi and degeneration of the internal organs in aged people or weak patients with chronic diseases.

2. Common diseases of the ear:

(1) *Furuncle in the external ear canal:*

Furuncle is often caused by injury or infection when removing ear wax. The patient may suffer from local pulsating pain, radiating to that side of the head, and the pain may be severe enough to interfere with sleep. There may also be swelling of the external canal, impairment of hearing, general malaise and low fever.

(2) *Inflammation of the external ear canal:*

The etiology of inflammation is same as that of furuncle in the external canal. At the early stage, only some congestion can be found in the deep part of the ear canal, and then diffuse redness, swelling, thickening, severe pain, erosion of skin with thin pus, general malaise and higher fever may appear.

(3) *Otitis media:*

This disease can be divided into the acute and chronic, and suppurative or non-suppurative types caused by obstruction of the auditory tube, allergic reaction and inflammation. The patient may suffer from a blocking sensation in the ear, deafness, tinnitus, hallucinations and thickening of the opaque ear drum membrane, accumulation of pus in the middle ear, fever, annoyance and poor appetite; vomiting and diarrhea may occur in children with this disease.

3. Inspection of the ears and diagnosis of diseases:

The ear is the external orifice of the kidneys. According to traditional Chinese medical theory: "Kidney qi can be supplied to the ear, and the ear can hear different sounds if the kidneys are healthy." Therefore, the ear can display diseases of the internal organs and external structure of body through the linkage of meridians with them. As a simple method of diagnosis, the inspection of the shape and color of the ear auricle by the naked eye can help in the diagnosis of diseases.

As a useful information, the projecting areas of various internal organs and different parts of the body on the ear are shown in the following figure (Fig. 3-2)

(1) *Inspection of the color of the ear auricle and diagnosis of diseases:*

The ears of a normal person should be light yellow in color, with a red tinge.

The bluish purple color of ear auricles is due to fright, epilepsy, attack of heat pathogens or invasion of wind-cold pathogens into the abdomen causing colic pain; bluish black color may appear in patients with pain due to deficiency of kidney water or production of fire pathogens from cold kidney water; pure black color may appear in patients with excessive disease of the kidneys or exhaustion of kidney qi; light black color may appear in patients with deficient diseases of the kidneys; charred black color indicates deficient heat pathogens in the kidneys, deficiency of kidney essence, water, Yin and qi or Xiaxiao (lower type of diabetes mellitus); and dirty charred color indicates bone diseases.

White color of ear auricles may appear in patients with cold and deficient syndrome caused by attack of wind-cold

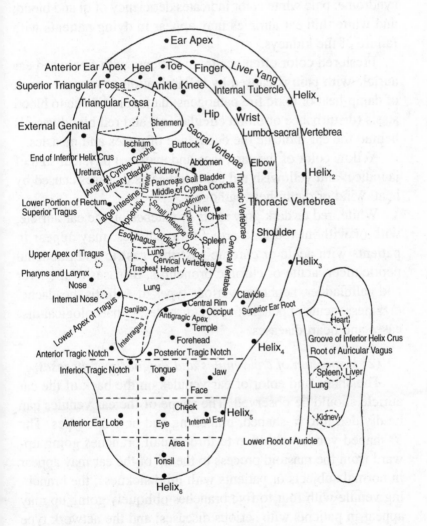

Fig. 3-2 Correlation between the ear and the different parts of the body

pathogens; bluish white color indicates a deficient cold syndrome; pale white color indicates deficiency of qi and blood; and white thin ear auricles may appear in dying patients with failure of the kidneys.

Fresh red color often occurs in patients with fever; red ear auricle with pain is caused by inflammation or upward attack of damp-heat or toxic fire pathogens; dark color is due to blood stasis (disturbance of blood circulation); and red blood vessels behind the ear indicate the occurence of poxes and measles.

Yellow color of the ears, face and eyes is a physical sign of jaundice; and yellowish red color indicates diseases caused by heat, wind or damp-heat pathogens.

White, red or dark grey spots or patches on the ear auricle, with or without red halo around the patches, may appear in patients with acute or chronic gastritis, gastric and duodenal peptic ulcer, acute or chronic bronchitis, diseases of the liver and gallbladder, nephritis, various types of arthritis, headache, dizziness, acute appendicitis, eye diseases, gynaecological diseases and heart diseases.

(2) *Inspection of ear venules and diagnosis of diseases:*
The shape and color of ear venules on the back of the ear auricle should be observed. The shape of the ear venules can be divided into Y-shaped, branching and network types. The Y-shaped venule with two to three small branches going upward from the mastoid process to the tip of the ear may appear in normal subjects or patients with mild sickness; the branching venule with four to five branches obliquely going up may appear in patients with serious diseases; and the network type of venule, like a spider's web without apparent main trunk, may appear in patients with critical diseases. Red venule indicates

attack of heat pathogens to the external and internal organs; blue venule indicates attack of wind pathogens and stagnation of qi and blood; purple venule indicates accumulation of heat pathogens in the body; and black venule indicates accumulation of cold pathogens in the body. In general, red venules may appear in patients with mild diseases, purple venules in patients with severe diseases and black venules in patients with critical diseases.

(3) *Inspection of shape of ear and diagnosis of diseases:*

Big and thick ear indicates sufficiency of kidney qi, and small and thin ear indicates deficiency of kidney qi.

Dry scaly ear helix indicates intestinal abscess or appears in chronic patients with blood stasis; and dry, thin and withered helix in a dark red color indicates extreme deficiency of vital energy, deficiency of kidney essence or exhaustion of kidney Yin.

Red swollen ear auricle indicates wind-heat pathogens in Shangjiao (upper energizer), excessive fire pathogens in the liver and gallbladder; hyperplasia of cartilage in more than two foci on the ear auricle is an indication of cancer; a small digital depression on the back of the ear auricle may appear in patients with congenital hypogenesis of the nervous system or in people susceptible to schizophrenia.

A small cherry-shaped nodule may appear in the external auditory meatus. A fresh red ear indicates accumulation of heat pathogens in the liver and gallbladder or attack of toxic heat pathogens to the ear; a light red ear indicates deficiency of the spleen and kidneys; and a dark red ear indicates long-lasting stagnation of toxic pathogens in the body or stagnation of qi and blood.

61

Purplish red or bluish purple ear helix with erosion is due to frostbite.

(4) *Inspection of excreta from ear meatus and diagnosis of diseases:*

Chronic discharge of pus from a withered ear with deviation of mouth and eyes is caused by excessive toxic pathogens or deficiency of qi and blood; and discharge of pus from the ear, with headache, vomiting, fever, coma, convulsions and stiff neck may appear in patients with Huanger Shanghan (otitis media with intracranial infection).

Patients with Erchuang (infection of the external auditory meatus) may suffer from diffuse redness, swelling, ulceration and exudation of external meatus. Patients with this disease, with fever, chills, headache and general malaise are attacked by wind and toxic heat pathogens; and patients with radiating pain to the temporal region and brain, bitter taste in the mouth, dryness in the throat, fever, chills, constipation and passage of dark urine are suffering from upward attack of damp-heat pathogens from the liver and gallbladder.

Patients with Xuanerfeng (eczema of the ear) may suffer from phagus behind the ear, and redness, erosion, exudate, hotness, itching and pain on and around the ear auricle with some general symptoms such as fever and annoyance; and severe Xuanerfeng with much yellow discharge is caused by attack of wind and damp-heat pathogens.

Repeated relapses of discharge of foul purulent pus from the ear over a long period of time is due to attack of external wind and damp-heat pathogens; foul discharge like putrefied cheese is due to deficiency of the kidneys and upward attack of damp-heat pathogens; and putrefaction of flesh and bone in the ear is due to excess pathogens and deficiency of vital energy (impairment of body resistance).

III. Inspection of the Nose and Diagnosis of Diseases

1. Inspection of the shape of the nose and diagnosis of diseases:

Black or brown spots or patches on the skin of the nose bridge are due to exposure to sunlight or pigmentation caused by other diseases, such as Kala-azar and liver diseases.

Red patch on the skin of the nose bridge with the lesion elevated over the surrounding normal skin and bilaterally spread to the cheeks may appear in patients with systemic lupus erythematosus; and red thickened patch with telangiectasis on the tip and alae of the nose may appear in acne rosacea (brandy nose).

Deformed nose with broad and flat nose bridge, like a frog's, and complete blockage of the nasal cavities may appear in patients with nasal polyps; and saddle nose is caused by the destruction and depression of the nose in patients with fracture or hypoplasia of the nasal bones or congenital syphilis.

Nostrils which dilate during inhalation and retract during exhalation may appear in patients with dyspnea and high fever, bronchial asthma or cardiac asthma.

The acute swelling of nasal mucosa with nasal obstruction and running nose is caused by inflammation and congestion in a case of acute rhinitis; chronic thickening of nasal mucosa may occur in chronic rhinitis of different etiology; and patients with chronic atrophic rhinitis may suffer from decreased nasal discharge, dryness, shrunken nasal conchae, dilated nasal cavities and impairment or absence of sense of smell.

Deviation of the nose or vertical wrinkles on the nose indicate poor heart function; deviation of the nasal septum indicates scoliosis of the spinal column; and roughness, pink color and lusterlessness of bilateral nasal alae and the philtrum region indicate dysfunction of the stomach and intestines or persistent constipation.

Patients with mongolism may have soft nose tip, constant protrusion of the tongue from the mouth, dull complexion and wide distance between the eyes.

Breathing through the mouth and speaking with a twang may appear in patients with nasal obstruction or chronic rhinitis.

Depression of the nose bridge and loss of eyebrows may appear in patients with severe leprosy.

In the early stage of nasal furuncle, a millet-like lesion with a pointed tip, a small white pustule and a red, swollen, hard and painful induration appears on the nose.

Nasal bleeding may occur in one or both nostrils. Unilateral nasal bleeding may occur in patients with external trauma, infection of the nasal cavity, injury to local blood vessels, tumor in the nasal cavity or deviation of the nasal septum; and bilateral nasal bleeding may occur in general diseases of the whole body, such as febrile infectious diseases, blood diseases, hypertensive disease, avitaminosis of C or K, and diseases of the liver and spleen. Periodic nasal bleeding may appear in women with endometriosis.

In ancient times, it was thought that a person with a high and straight nose and upright and big nose bulb would have a long life, while a person with a small and withered nose would have a short life span.

2. Inspection of the color of the nose and diagnosis of diseases:

The normal nose is bright, and the nasal mucosa is pink and shiny.

White nose bulb indicates deficiency of qi and blood or depletion of blood. It may appear in children with diarrhea and indigestion due to deficiency of the spleen; white nose may appear in patients with diseases of the lungs with cold sputum or chronic bronchitis; pale nasal mucosa indicates a cold syndrome; flushed mucosa indicates accumulation of endogenous heat pathogens; blue nose bulb indicates diseases of the stomach and intestines with abdominal pain, which is more severe in patients with cold nose bulb; bluish black nose in children indicates a critical disease or severe pain caused by cold pathogens; bluish yellow nose in a dull face indicates liver disease; and bluish yellow nose bulb often appears in patients with stranguria.

Red nose bulb indicates excessive heat pathogens in the lungs and spleen; light red nose bulb indicates deficient heat pathogens in the spleen; red nose alae in women indicate amenorhea; children with reddish purple nose bridge are susceptible to furuncles and other lesions with pus and blood; fresh red nose may appear in patients with polycythemia; patients with red nose and dry nasal cavity are susceptible to nasal bleeding; congested nose scattered with blood streaks (dilated capillary vessels) often appears on the bluish yellow face of patients with cirrhosis of the liver; and red swollen nostrils indicate diseases caused by toxic heat pathogens.

Yellow nose bulb indicates accumulation of damp-heat pathogens in the body or cold pathogens in the chest; cold pathogens may cause diseases of the colon with poor appetite and constipation; bright deep yellow nose indicates blood stasis; and yellowish black withered nose indicates fire pathogens in the spleen and exhaustion of body fluid.

A light black nose bulb indicates accumulation of water in the body; black withered nose may appear in patients suffering from over-indulgence in sexual activity; black nose alae indicate pain in the abdomen; black nose alae with black philtrum indicates pain in the testes and penis; black nose alae in women indicate diseases with pain in the urinary bladder and uterus; black nose alae with black philtrum indicate disturbance of leukorrhea and lochia in women; dry coal-black nostrils indicate deep invasion of toxic heat pathogens, accumulation of dryness and heat pathogens in the colon or lung failure; black and shiny nose bulb indicates intake of too much improper food; blue and cold nose indicates a critical disease with exhaustion of lung and stomach qi; sweat droplets on the nose bulb indicate severe pain in the heart and abdomen; the appearance of coal-black nose indicates a very bad prognosis; the diseases of patients with a shiny and moist nose on a black face are still curable, but they are difficult to cure if the nose is withered; children with bluish black nose bridge may suffer from a serious disease; extraordinarily wide or narrow distance between the eyes indicates heart failure or deformity of the heart; extremely small nose with a very narrow nose bridge in women indicates abnormality of the heart; and deviated nose or vertical wrinkles on the nose indicates weakness of the internal organs.

3. Inspection of the nose bridge of children and diagnosis of diseases:

The inspection of the nose bridge (region between the inner canthi of the eyes) in children is more convenient and useful than that of finger venules for the diagnosis of diseases. The inspection of nose bridge includes the observation of color, depth and direction of superficial venules in this region. Abnormal findings in this region are closely related to diseases of the respiratory and digestive systems.

Common colors of the nose bridge in children are blue, yellow and red. Blue color indicates diseases of the digestive system, with diarrhea, vomiting, indigestive malnutrition, abdominal pain and poor appetite; yellow color indicates malnutrition, avitaminosis or dysentery; and red color indicates diseases of the respiratory system, including upper respiratory infection, bronchitis, asthma and pneumonia.

The direction of the venules of the nose bridge may be vertical, oblique or horizontal. Vertical venules indicate respiratory diseases, such as bronchitis and upper respiratory infection. The diagnosis of diseases in children with oblique venules can be made only after evaluation of information obtained by this method and other diagnosis methods. Engorged venules on the nose bridge indicate chronic diseases.

The color of the venules of the nose bridge is usually similar to that of those between the eyebrows, behind the outer canthi of the eyes, at the corners of the forehead and in the nasolabial grooves. Blue engorged venules on the nose bridge and the area between the eyebrows indicate diarrhea, or fright and convulsions; blue engorged venules on the nose bridge and at the corners of the forehead may appear in patients with fright due to heat pathogens in the gallbladder; and yellow venules on the nose bridge and in the nasolabial grooves indicate stomach stagnation and injury to the spleen.

Chapter 4

INSPECTION OF THE ORAL CAVITY AND PHILTRUM, AND DIAGNOSIS OF DISEASES

The mouth is an external orifice of the spleen, and the lips are the external structure related to the spleen. As traditional physicians put it: "The mouth and lips are related structures of the spleen." The function of the mouth and lips is to take in water and food, secrete saliva and speak. Therefore, the mouth and lips can show the condition of all internal organs and meridians, including the spleen and stomach, because they are the important communications gate of the internal organs and a key pivot of human life.

The teeth are exposed parts of the bone structure, and the gums are connected to the stomach. They are closely connected with the internal organs through several meridians, and the essence and qi of the internal organs can be transported through these meridians to nourish them for preserving the health of the gums and consolidating the teeth. Then the teeth and gums can normally play their roles in grinding food, improving digestion and assisting phonation. Otherwise, the gums may become atrophic, and the teeth may be lost if the essence and qi of the internal organs is depleted.

The throat is a gate of the lungs and stomach, and a communications pass of breath and intake of food. It is connected with many internal organs, first of all, the lungs, stomach and kidneys, through several meridians and shows their pathological changes.

It is well known that the tongue is a mirror of disease. Inspection of the tongue can show the condition of the internal organs, the nature of pathogens and the severity of disease, because it is closely connected with the meridians of all internal organs. It is particularly useful in the diagnosis of diseases of the digestive, circulatory and nervous systems. Both the tongue proper and the tongue coating should be carefully observed.

I. Inspection of the Lips and Diagnosis of Diseases

The lips of normal people should be bright red in color, because they have numerous capillary vessels. Because of the emptiness of the capillary vessels and decrease of hemoglobin in the blood, the lips may turn pale in patients with fainting, aortic incompetence or anemia; dark red lips are due to promotion of blood circulation or engorgement of capillary vessels in patients of acute febrile diseases; and cynotic lips are due to increase of reduced hemoglobin in blood in patients with dysfunction of the heart and lungs.

Dry lips with fissures may appear in patients with severe dehydration; clusters of small vesicles on the boundary of the skin and mucosa of the lips may appear in patients with herpes of the lips caused by herpes simplex virus as a common clinical manifestation of lobar pneumonia, influenza, epiedmic cerebrospinal meningitis or malaria.

The sudden appearance of non-inflammatory swelling of the

69

lips is known as angioneurotic edema; erosion of the mouth angles may appear in deficiency of riboflavin; and large thick lips may appear in patients of cretinism, myxedema and acromegaly.

(1) *Change of color of the lips:*
The inspection of the color of the lips is similar to that of facial color. The change of lip color is more remarkable because the mucosa of the lips is thin and transparent, and the inspection of lip color is therefore more convenient.

Normal red and moist lips indicate sufficiency of stomach qi and balance of qi and blood; thick red lips in women indicate fullness of Chongmai (thoroughfare vessel) and smooth delivery of a baby; fresh red lips indicate deficiency of Yin and excessiveness of fire pathogens; dark red lips indicate excessive heat syndrome; dry dark red lips indicate depletion of body fluid and excessiveness of heat pathogens in the body; dry crimson lips with fissures indicate invasion of heat pathogens into Ying (nutrient component) and blood; and vermilion red lips in chronic patients indicate a bad prognosis due to floating of deficient Yang over the body surface.

Lips as pale as white paper and surrounded by white borders indicate exhaustion of blood; and pale lips in pregnant women due to deficiency of blood may indicate difficult delivery.

Pale lips with black tint indicate accumulation of cold pathogens in the body, and bluish black lips indicate excessive accumulation of cold pathogens in the body; apoplectic patients with bluish black color below the nose, foamy spittle from the mouth and rigid body may die soon; blue lips in patients with tremor of the limbs and slight sweating indicate liver failure;

bluish black lips or blue lips on a black face indicate death; deathly black lips indicate extreme deficiency of qi and blood; black lips in patients with extremely cold body and limbs also indicate death, due to invasion of pathogens into the solid internal organs; and blue lips in patients with warm body and sweating indicate a mild disease due to invasion of pathogens into the hollow organs, and the disease may be cured soon.

Black philtrum in patients with diarrhea and sudden onset of severe pain in the lower abdomen is a sign of bad prognosis; vermilion red lips in patients with severe diarrhea are also a critical sign; light red color in the philtrum indicates diseases with pain; light black color in the philtrum indicates a heat syndrome; blue color in the philtrum indicates a cold syndrome, and white color in the philturm indicates a critical disease difficult to cure.

(2) *Change of shape of lips:*
Dry lips with fissures indicate deficiency of body fluid due to attack of external heat and dryness pathogens, wasting of body fluid by heat pathogens or accumulation of heat pathogens in the spleen.

Dripping of saliva from the side of the mouth indicates deficiency of the spleen and excessiveness of dampness pathogens or accumulation of heat pathogens in the stomach; it often occurs in children with deviation and incomplete closure of the mouth due to attack of wind pathogens.

Locked jaw and difficult sucking milk may appear in newborn babies with tetanus; blue pouted lips in children with uncontrollable convulsions is due to invasion of liver wind to the spleen; locked jaw may also appear in children with toxic dysentery.

A patient with the mouth always open is suffering from a deficiency syndrome; a patient with the mouth always open, like a fish, is suffering from spleen failure; and a patient with mouth open to exhale air but without apparent inhalation of air is suffering from lung failure.

Curled swollen upper lip with a flat philtrum in chronic or critical patients indicates exhaustion of spleen Yang; curled and retracted upper lip with a shortened philtrum incapable of covering the teeth indicates exhaustion of spleen Yin; and apoplectic patients with the mouth always open are suffering from exhaustion of heart qi.

White lichenoid ulcers in the oral cavity are due to excessiveness of Yang and deficiency of Yin, accumulation of damp-heat pathogens in the spleen or steaming up and sweltering by heat pathogens; naked lesions are painful and red in color after the white membranous covering is removed; oral aphthae are red, swollen and painful ulcers formed after rupture of the small white vesicles along the border of the lips, which are caused by the upward scorching of heat pathogens accumulated in the heart and spleen; fresh red erosive patches are produced by excessive fire pathogens; pink patches are produced by deficient fire pathogens; and snow-white patches all over the mouth cavity of young babies is known as thrush (mycotic stomatitis) and is caused by heat pathogens in the heart and spleen retained from the fetus.

Red, swollen and itching lips with burning pain and discharge from the fissures is known as Chunfeng (exfoliative inflammation of the lips), and is caused by upward invasion of fire pathogens in the stomach; a nodule in the size of a bean on the lip may gradually grow in size to form a hard and painful mass like a silkworm cocoon, known as Chunjian (lip cancer), and is caused by upward invasion of heat pathogens with phlegm from the stomach to lips. Small white spots on the labial frenum of the upper lip indicate the presence of hemorrhoids.

II. Inspection of Teeth and Gums, and Diagnosis of Diseases

1. Inspection of teeth and diagnosis of diseases:

Clean white and shiny teeth indicate sufficiency of body fluid and abundance of kidney qi or sufficient preservation of body fluid; dry yellow teeth may appear in patients with epidemic febrile diseases at the late stage or in patients with wasting of body fluid caused by excessive heat pathogens; teeth as dry as rocks indicate the presence of excessive heat pathogens in the stomach; and teeth as dry as dead bones indicate exhaustion of kidney Yin. In brief, dry teeth always indicate depletion of essence in the body.

The grinding of teeth as a prodromal sign of convulsions is due to the stirring up of wind by damp-heat pathogens or rushing past of qi through meridians due to heat pathogens in the stomach; the grinding of teeth in patients with deficiency syndrome and weak pulse is due to deficiency of stomach qi, and poor nourishment of muscles and blood vessels; lockjaw is due to blockage of collaterals by wind phlegm or stirring up of wind by excessive heat pathogens; and the grinding of teeth during sleep is due to accumulation of food or heat pathogens in the body.

Exposed loose teeth may appear in patients with kidney deficiency or upward flaming of deficient fire pathogens; re-

73

tarded eruption of permanent teeth after the loss of milk teeth in children is due to deficiency of calcium or weakness of the body; yellow, dry and loose teeth or abnormal loss of teeth in patients with severe diseases indicate bone decay; erosion of gums and loss of teeth is a critical sign of Yagan (ulcerative gingivitis); broken and loose teeth caused by external trauma are known as Douchi (fight tooth); and decayed teeth due to caries are due to tooth erosion caused by food debris retained between the teeth.

The teeth are closely related to the stomach, and the dental hygiene is often impaired by diseases of the stomach. The yellowish brown color of mottled teeth is due to drinking water high in fluorine content; and a crescent moon-shaped defect at the cutting edge of the incisors and splits between separated teeth may appear in patients of congenital syphilis.

2. Inspection of the gums and diagnosis of diseases:

The normal gum is pink in color, firm and closely attached to the neck of the tooth.

Edematous gum may appear in cases of chronic periodontitis; bleeding along the border of the gum often appears in patients of scurvy, blood diseases and hemorrhagic diseases; and bluish grey spots and line along the free border of the gums is called a lead line and is a physical sign of lead poisoning.

Pale gum indicates deficiency of blood to supply the gums; pale and atrophic gum is due to deficiency of stomach Yin; and red swollen gums are caused by upward flaming of stomach fire pathogens.

Bleeding from red, swollen and painful gums is due to damage to blood vessels by stomach heat pathogens; and bleeding from slightly swollen gums without redness and pain is due to deficiency of qi or damage to blood vessels by kidney fire pathogens.

Red, swollen and ulcerated gums with severe local pain, foul bloody discharge, chills and fever may appear in patients with ulcerated gingivitis due to invasion of toxic wind-heat pathogens to the stomach.

Red atrophic gums with ulcerated border is due to deficiency of kidney Yin and upward flaming of deficient fire pathogens; and formation of Chiyong (gingival papilla) from the gums is caused by irritant food.

III. Inspection of the Throat and Diagnosis of Diseases

The normal throat is pink in color, moist and smooth, without swelling or pain, and functions for breathing, phonation and the swallowing of food.

Red throat indicates accumulation of heat pathogens in the lungs and stomach; fresh red throat indicates deficiency of the lung and kidney Yin, and excessiveness of fire pathogens; white dry throat with thirst and slight pain, exacerbated by swallowing saliva is due to deficiency of qi and Yin; white, lusterless and swollen throat in patients with feeble pulse indicates a critical condition with floating of Yang over the body surface and vanishing of the spirit into the void; dark red and diffusely swollen throat indicates coagulation of phlegm and turbid fluid, and stagnation of qi and blood; pale throat indicates a deficient cold syndrome; red, swollen and ulcerated throat may appear in patients with excess syndrome; scattered superficial erosion in the throat may appear in patients with mild heat pathogens in the lungs and stomach; deep ulcers diffusely scattered in the throat indicate accumulation of violent heat pathogens; chronic ulceration with peripheral pink or pale borders may appear in deficiency syndrome; scattered superficial ulcers are due to upward flaming of deficient fire pathogens, and diffuse and deep ulceration is due to deficiency of qi, blood and kidney Yin or deep invasion of toxic pathogens.

Local red, soft and prominent swelling in the throat with fluctuation and depression under pressure is a mature abscess; if it is a hard mass, the abscess is still immature. Yellow sticky pus drained from the abscess indicates excessive syndrome; and thin and dirty pus may be drained from the abscess in patients with poor body resistance to overcome the pathogens. In patients with sufficient vital energy and good body resistance the pus can be drained off easily and the lesion can quickly heal; pus can not be easily drained away and lesions can not quickly heal in patients with deficiency of vital energy and poor body resistance.

Ulcerated lesions of the throat may be covered with a white pseudomembrane. If the pseudomembrane is thick, loose and easily peeled off, and no new membrane regenerates after it is removed, the lesions are caused by heat pathogens in the stomach; and in the case of severe diseases, such as diphtheria, the membrane is difficult to peel away, the forcible removal of the membrane may cause bleeding and a new membrane may regenerate after the original one is removed. Such lesions may appear in patients with exhaustion of Yin due to toxic heat pathogens in the lungs and stomach.

The induration, ulceration, necrosis or formation of pseudomembrane may appear in the throat and on the tonsils

76

of patients with agranulocytosis, leukemia and infectious mononucleosis.

Hoarse voice is an early symptom of vocal fold cancer or supraglottic cancer near the vocal fold. The early symptoms are not remarkable in patients with infraglottic cancer, and they may have only some discomfort and the sensation of a foreign body in the throat, but hoarse voice is a late symptom of this tumor.

Superficial ulceration and infection of cancer may cause pain radiating to the ear and blood in the sputum. Late cancer of the larynx may cause aphonia, pus and blood in the sputum, enlarged cervical lymph nodes, dyspnea, dysphagia, remote metastasis of tumor, general weakness and cachexia.

IV. Detection of Voice and Diagnosis of Diseases

The lungs, larynx, glottis, tongue, teeth, lips and nose contribute to produce the voice. The lungs are the source of energy to drive air for the production of the voice; the larynx is an organ of phonation to produce the voice, and the other organs adjust the voice. Change of voice can show the condition of the internal organs.

1. Voice of healthy subjects:

The voice of normal subjects is natural, harmonious, and in a proper tone and pitch. The voice of normal people may also be varied in accordance with their heredity and physical build. The voice of men is loud and dull; the voice of women is high and clear; the voice of children is sharp and crisp; and the voice of aged people is deep and raucous. At the same time, the voice can also be affected by emotional change. The varia-

77

tions of the voice mentioned above are still a modification within the normal range of the human voice.

2. Pathological voice:

The five musical notes of Jue (mi), Zhi (sou), Gong (dou), Shang (ri) and Yu (la) and the five modes of shouting, laughing, singing, crying and sighing are correlated with the five internal organs of the liver, heart, spleen, lungs and kidneys.

Hoarseness and aphonia: Patients with mild injury of the phonation organs may have hoarseness, and patients with severe injury may have no voice at all. Hoarseness and aphonia in cases of acute diseases caused by attack of external wind-cold or wind-heat pathogens may appear in patients with excess syndrome; hoarseness and aphonia may appear in chronic patients with deficiency syndrome with depletion of essence, deficiency of lung and kidney Yin, and exhaustion of fluid in the lungs due to attack of deficient fire pathogens in the lungs; shouting in fury may produce hoarseness after injury to the larynx; and aphonia in pregnant women is due to blockage of upward transportation of kidney essence by the fetus.

Snoring during sleep is a physiological phenomenon caused by partial blockage of the respiratory tract, so that it is not a pathological voice; but continuous loud snoring may appear in critical patients of apoplexy (stroke) with coma, flaccid limbs and incontinence of urine due to damage of internal solid organs.

Continuous moaning indicates pain or distension in the body; moaning in patients with the eyebrows knitted indicates headache; moaning of bedridden patients indicates pain in the waist and legs; moaning in patients who press their heart or abdomen with the palm indicates pain in the chest or abdomen;

and moaning in patients who press the cheek with the palm indicates toothache.

Sudden shouting by quiet people indicates diseases of the bones or joints; speaking in a feeble voice indicates diseases of the heart or diaphragm; repeated sharp screaming with a frightening expression indicates convulsions; and night crying by children indicates diseases caused by fright, heat pathogens in the heart or spleen, or abdominal pain due to cold pathogens in the spleen.

Speaking in a loud and monotonous voice, with the volume gradually increased indicates diseases due to attack of external pathogens; speaking in a low and weak voice with the volume gradually decreasing indicates deficient diseases due to injury to the internal organs; endless talking in a high and loud voice in patients with annoyance indicates excessive heat syndrome; occasional speaking by taciturn people in a low and soft voice indicates a deficient cold syndrome; muttering to oneself stopped by the appearance of a stranger is called Duyu (murmur); incoherent and irrational talking is called Cuoyu (talking nonsense). They all indicate a deficient syndrome due to deficiency of heart qi and wandering of the mind.

Short breathing with quick and short respiration can be divided into deficient and excessive types. The deficient type is due to deficiency of lung qi, and the excessive type is due to accumulation of phlegm and rheum in the body or adverse ascent of qi.

Rough breathing is due to invasion of excessive pathogens from outside, and weak breathing indicates deficiency of vital energy (impairment of body resistance). In patients with normal breathing the disease is limited to the organic structures of the body with qi (function) not affected; but both organic structures and qi are simultaneously damaged in patients with abnormal breath.

Asthma with quick and short breaths and dyspnea can be divided into deficient and excessive types. The prompt onset of asthma of excessive type in patients with rough and rushing breath to release chest distress, upward tilted head, protruded eyes, robust physique and full and forceful pulse is due to excessive heat pathogens in the lungs and accumulation of phlegm and rheum in the body; patients of the Xiao (excessive) type may have quick and short breath with an intermittent high-pitched whistling noise in the throat caused by accumulation of phlegm and rheum in the body and induced by attack of external cold pathogens to body surface. Cold and damp living environment and intake of sour, cold or uncooked food are also factors leading to asthma.

3. Evaluation of cough and diagnosis of diseases:

The cough is a common symptom of lung diseases. A muffled cough indicates a disease caused by cold and dampness pathogens; a loud and dull cough with white, clear and thin sputum and nasal obstruction indicates a disease caused by attack of external wind and cold pathogens; and a low-sounding cough with profuse sputum easily expectorated is caused by cold and dampness pathogens or accumulation of phlegm and rheum.

A clear and crisp cough is caused by heat and dryness pathogens; and a dry cough with a small amount of sticky sputum or without sputum is caused by fire, heat or dryness pathogens.

A low and weak cough in patients with shortness of breath and expectoration of white foamy sputum is due to deficiency of the lungs; night cough is due to deficiency of kidney water; and cough in the early morning is due to deficiency of the spleen or accumulation of cold and dampness pathogens in the colon.

Acute cough with a hoarse voice indicates an excess syndrome; a chronic cough with a hoarse voice indicates a deficiency syndrome due to damage to the internal organs; a dull cough in patients with yellow sticky sputum difficult to spit out, dryness and pain in the throat and hot breath from the nose is due to heat pathogens in the lungs; and a muffled cough indicates poor dispersion of lung qi.

Paroxysmal attacks of continuous coughing with whooping like the cry of an egret may appear in children with whooping cough caused by attack of wind pathogens and blockage of the air passage by phlegm; and a cough like the barking of a dog may appear in patients with diphtheria.

Sneezing produced by the rushing of air through the nose usually appears in cases of common cold caused by wind-cold pathogens; and sneezing in cases of chronic diseases due to accumulation of external pathogens on the body surface indicates a good prognosis of the disease.

In modern medicine the cough is considered as a protective reflex of respiratory system occurring in many diseases, such as tracheitis, bronchitis, pulmonary tuberculosis, emphysema of the lungs and lung cancer.

The cough can be divided into two types — with or without sputum. A dry choking cough may appear in patients with acute bronchitis, endobronchial tuberculosis, chronic laryngopharygitis, lung cancer or pleuritis.

A cough with sputum may appear in patients of chronic bronchitis, bronchiectasis, pneumonia and pulmonary tuberculosis; severe paroxysmal cough may appear in patients with foreign body in the bronchus, bronchial tuberculosis and in veteran smokers; and persistent cough may appear in patients of pulmonary tuberculosis and chronic bronchitis.

Cough with fever may appear in patients with infection of the respiratory tract and pleuritis; cough with hemoptysis may appear in patients of bronchiectasis, pulmonary tuberculosis and lung cancer; cough with chest pain may appear in patients with lobar pneumonia and pleuritis; cough with pathological leanness may appear in patients of pulmonary tuberculosis or lung cancer; cough with asthma may appear in patients with bronchial asthma, cardiogenic asthma, asthmatic bronchitis and foreign body in the bronchus; cough with palpitations of the heart may appear in patients of left heart failure with rapid pulse, orthopnea, continuous cough and expectoration of bloody foamy sputum; and cough with dyspnea may appear in patients with severe heart or lung diseases.

4. Evaluation of crying and laughing in children and diagnosis of diseases:

Crying in children can be divided into the physiological and pathological types: Physiological crying often occurs in hungry babies or in babies suffering from thirst, lack of sleep, improper clothes, wet diaper or needing for affection. Physiological crying is loud, and the spirit and complexion of babies should be normal in the interval between episodes of crying.

Pathological crying is usually caused by discomfort or suffering in a certain part of the body. The baby may have a sudden onset of crying, screaming and struggling with expression of distress, flexed limbs, clenched fists and frowning. Common causes of pathological crying are as follows:

(1) Rickets: Rickets is caused by deficiency of calcium and

vitamin D. Besides crying and struggling, the babies also have profuse sweating, fear, restlessness, sparse hair, enlarged fontanel, chicken breast and frog belly.

(2) Thrush: Thrush usually occurs in infants with poor nutrition and weak body. The mouth cavity is edematous, congested and covered with white membrane, and the excretion of saliva is increased.

(3) Acute tonsillitis: The babies may cry and struggle endlessly with fever, and refuse to suck milk because of sore throat.

(4) Meningitis: The babies may constantly cry, scream and struggle because of headache due to increase of intracranial pressure with bulging fontanel, staring eyes, stiff neck, rigid limbs and fear of elevating and rotating the head.

(5) Abdominal pain: The babies may suddenly cry following the onset of abdominal pain and stop crying after relief of abdominal pain. At the same time, they may also have a pale complexion, cold sweats, vomiting, diarrhea, hematochezia and palpable mass in the abdomen. Palpation of the abdomen always causes crying. Abdominal pain may occur in cases of acute inflammation of the intestines, intestinal obstruction, indigestion, intestinal parasites and appendicitis.

(6) Diseases of the ear: Acute otitis media with fever may be caused by accidental dropping of milk into the external meatus of the ear, and the babies may endlessly cry and struggle, especially when the ear auricle is pressed; and babies with furuncle in the external meatus of the ear or acute parotitis may also have fever, local swelling and refusal to palpate over the lesion.

(7) Anal fissure, infection of the urinary tract, eczema and hookworm disease may also cause crying and struggling in babies.

Healthy and intelligent babies always show a smiling face, and the disappearance of smiling indicates the deterioration of disease in a sick baby. The occurrence of an apathic, suffering and dull expression after the disappearance of smiling over one day indicates severe sickness in babies.

V. Inspection of the Philtrum and Beard, and Diagnosis of Diseases

1. Inspection of the philtrum:

The Renzhong acupoint (GV 26) lies in the philtrum, at a junction of its upper one third and lower two-thirds. A stiff and flat philtrum indicates the swelling of the throat and rigidity of the neck and shoulder.

A slightly flat philtrum and stiff upper lip in patients with bright and soft lower lip indicates a susceptibility to skin rashes and vesicles on the hand, foot and face.

A white philtrum and dark red right upper lip indicate abdominal distension and pain due to damp-heat in the stomach and deficient cold pathogens in the colon; and a white philtrum and light white upper and lower lips indicate pain in the waist, shoulder and back, and abdominal distension due to accumulation of cold pathogens in the colon, small intestine and abdominal cavity.

Stiffness and depression in the left or right part of the philtrum indicate poor circulatory function of the left or right abdominal cavity; and stiffness, swelling and darkness of the left (or right) part of the philtrum indicate susceptibility to malignant diseases in the left (or right) abdominal cavity.

A faint blue color in the philtrum of a woman indicates

dysmenorrhea; a flushing red color in the lower part of the philtrum of a woman indicates profuse uterine bleeding due to heat pathogens in the blood; and a pale white color on the upper part of the philtrum of a woman indicates profuse uterine bleeding due to deficiency of qi.

A blackish blue color on the philtrum of a man indicates orchitis and prostatitis with pain; and a pale and shallow philtrum in men indicates susceptibility to impotence and emission of semen.

2. Inspection of beard:

A long, shiny and soft beard indicates plentiful qi and blood in the stomach meridian; a short beard indicates plentiful qi and scanty blood in the stomach meridian; a sparse beard indicates plentiful blood and scanty qi in the stomach meridian; absence of beard indicates scanty qi and blood in the stomach meridian; and shiny body hair indicates deficiency of qi in the spleen and stomach.

VI. Inspection of the Tongue and Diagnosis of Diseases

1. Normal tongue:

The normal tongue is "pink in color with a thin white coating." The tongue proper should be soft, flexible in movement, pink in color, fresh and shiny in appearance and proper in thickness without deformity. A thin white coating composed of fine granules is evenly spread over the tongue, with proper moisture, but it is not sticky and greasy. The coating can not be erased from the tongue.

2. Relation between the tongue and the internal organs:

The tongue is divided into the tip, center, root and borders for inspection, to make diagnosis of diseases of the internal organs (Fig. 4-1).

The tip of the tongue can indicate diseases of the heart and lungs; the center can indicate diseases of the spleen and stomach; the root can indicate diseases of the kidneys and urinary bladder; and both borders can indicate diseases of the liver and gallbladder.

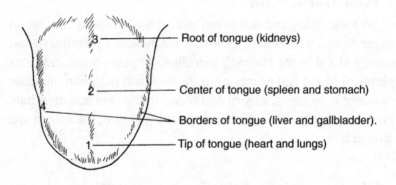

3 —— Root of tongue (kidneys)

2 —— Center of tongue (spleen and stomach)

—— Borders of tongue (liver and gallbladder).

1 —— Tip of tongue (heart and lungs)

Fig. 4-1   Areas of the internal organs reflected on the tongue

3. Methods, steps and cautions for inspection of the tongue:

(1) *Methods and steps:*

The patients should be asked to protrude the tongue naturally out of the mouth against a light source for full exposure. Changes in the tongue proper and the coating on the tip, center, root and borders of the tongue are observed.

(2) *Cautions:*

The tongue should be protruded naturally, without any tension; otherwise, the color of the tongue tip may turn redder than normal; it should be protruded flat, without rolling or twisting; and the protrusion of the tongue should not be held for a long interval; otherwise, it may turn darker in color.

The tongue should be observed in good natural light rather than lamplight, which may produce a misdiagnosis.

The intake of food may affect the appearance of the tongue: For example, water may turn the tongue more moist; intake of hot and spicy food may turn the tongue darker in color; intake of tangerine, Huanglian (goldthread rhizome) and riboflavine may stain the tongue yellow; black plums or olives may stain the tongue black; and the thickness of the tongue coating may be changed by chewing food.

There are also some variations of appearance of the tongue in normal subjects. For example, in obese people the tongue is bigger and the coating is slightly greasy; and in thin people the tongue is smaller and dark in color.

People who indulge in smoking, or taking alcohol or sour and spicy food may have a dark red tongue proper and yellow or greyish black tongue coating.

In the rainy season, the tongue coating is thicker; and in the dry season the tongue proper is dark red in color and the coating is slightly dry.

4. Items for inspection of the tongue:

For inspection of the tongue, both tongue proper and tongue coating should be observed. The tongue proper, also called the tongue body, is the freely movable muscular part of the tongue, and the tongue coating is the lichenoid covering on the tongue

87

proper.

The color and shape of the tongue can indicate the condition of the internal organs, and the quantity of qi and blood; and the tongue coating can show the location of lesions, nature of diseases and violence of pathogens.

(1) *Inspection of the tongue proper:*

1) Appearance of the tongue: The normal tongue proper should be red in color, vivid and bright in appearance; a dry and rigid tongue without luster and vitality indicates a critical disease.

2) Color of the tongue: The important variations of tongue color are as follows:

Pale tongue: A pale tongue is light red in color, paler than that of a normal pink tongue, or even completely colorless. A pale tongue indicates a deficient and cold syndrome due to deficiency of qi and blood, deficiency of Yang qi, reduction of formation of Yin and blood, and impairment of the blood circulation to supply blood to the tongue; a pale, moist, puffy and tender tongue proper indicates a cold syndrome due to deficiency of Yang; and a pale, bright, lean and thin tongue proper indicates deficiency of qi and blood.

Red tongue: A red tongue is fresh red in color, and darker than that of a normal pink tongue. This is due to promotion of blood circulation by excessive heat pathogens and congestion of blood vessels in the tongue. A red tongue indicates a heat syndrome; a fresh red tongue with prickles and yellow thick coating indicates an excessive heat syndrome; and a fresh red tongue with scanty coating and fissures or a bright red and naked tongue (without coating) indicates a deficient heat syndrome.

Crimson tongue: A crimson tongue is reddish purple in color, indicating diseases caused by external pathogens or internal injury. A crimson tongue with red spots or prickles indicates diseases caused by invasion of heat pathogens into Ying (nutrient) and blood in epidemic febrile diseases: Crimson tongue with scanty coating and fissures or bare crimson tongue is due to deficiency of Yin and excessiveness of fire pathogens in diseases due to internal injury; and moist crimson tongue with scanty coating is due to accumulation of cold pathogens and blood stasis.

Blue tongue: The color of a blue tongue is the same as that of engorged veins on the skin or similar to the color of a buffalo's tongue. It is caused by the dominance of cold pathogens, stagnation of Yang qi and stasis of blood. A blue color over the whole tongue indicates invasion of cold pathogens into the liver and kidneys, and stagnation of Yang qi; blue color along the border of the tongue with dryness in the mouth but without desire to drink water is due to blood stasis.

A blue or purple tint may occur in a tongue of any color mentioned above to give a dark appearance; it always indicates stagnation of qi and blood.

3) Shape of the tongue: The bulk, tenderness, puffiness and particular deformities of the tongue should be observed, which may be described as follows:

Tenderness: A tongue with a tough texture, coarse fissures and coating of any color indicates an excessive syndrome; and a tongue with a tender texture, puffy appearance and fine creases indicates a deficient syndrome.

Big tongue: A big and fat tongue, larger than that of normal subjects and occupying the whole oral cavity is due to accumulation and blockage of phlegm, rheum and dampness; a pale, fat and tender tongue with a slippery and watery coating indicates deficiency of spleen and kidney Yang, disturbance of metabolism and retention of body fluid; and a pink (or red), big and fat tongue with a yellow greasy coating is due to contention between turbid phlegm and damp-heat in the spleen and stomach or due to upward overflowing of damp-heat, phlegm and rheum.

Swollen tongue: A big swollen tongue filling the whole oral cavity and interfering with closure of the mouth may be produced by the following causes: A fresh red and swollen tongue with pain may appear in patients with heat pathogens in the heart and spleen, accumulation of heat in the blood vessels and upward overflowing of qi and blood; a purple swollen tongue may appear in alcoholics with febrile disease due to upward overflowing of heat pathogens and alcohol intoxication; and a dark bluish purple and swollen tongue may appear in patients with stasis and coagulation of blood due to intoxication. A purple swollen tongue may also appear in patients with congenital obstruction of the blood vessels of the tongue, such as the hemangioma of the tongue.

Thin tongue: A small thin tongue is caused by deficiency of qi, blood and Yin to fill up the tongue proper. A pale, lean and thin tongue is due to deficiency of qi and blood or deficiency of Yin and excessiveness of fire pathogens; and a dry, crimson, thin and lean tongue is due to deficiency of Yin, excessiveness of fire pathogens and depletion of body fluids.

Spots on the tongue: Scattered red, white or black bulging spots on the tongue is called Hongxingshe (red star tongue). The soft granules scattered over the tip and bilateral borders of the tongue may gradually grow in size to form elevated sharp prickles and to produce a pricking sensation to the palpating hand; and bluish purple or purplish black patches of varied size and irregular shape are called ecchymosis (bruise). Red, black and white spots on the tongue are all caused by excessive toxic heat pathogens, but red spots indicate invasion of toxic warm pathogens into the blood, attack of toxic heat pathogens to the heart and accumulation of damp-heat pathogens in the blood; the white spots as a preliminary lesion of erosion indicate deficiency of spleen and stomach qi and attack of toxic heat pathogens to Chongmai (thoroughfare vessel); and black spots indicate extreme excessiveness of heat pathogens in the blood and stagnation of qi and blood.

Prickles on the tongue: The formation of prickles on the tongue is due to accumulation of excessive heat pathogens in Sanjiao (triple energizer), qi component or Ying (nutrient) component. The prickles on a roasted yellow tongue coating are due to extreme excessiveness of heat pathogens in qi component; and the prickles on a bare crimson tongue are due to invasion of heat pathogens into Ying (nutrient) and blood, and depletion of Yin. Prickles on the tip of the tongue indicate excessiveness of heart fire pathogens; and prickles on the central area of the tongue indicate excessive heat pathogens in the stomach and intestines.

Fissures on the tongue: Fissures of different number, depth and shape are all due to deficiency of Yin and blood to nourish the surface of the tongue. They are short creases arranged in vertical, horizontal or radiating directions, or in gyral or cobble pattern. The fissures on the tongue may be due to exhaustion of Yin by excessive heat pathogens, deficiency of blood to moisten the tongue, or attack on deficient spleen by dampness pathogens; crimson tongue with fissures indicates exhaustion of body fluid by excessive heat pathogens or deficiency of Yin and depletion of body fluids; pale white tongue with fissures indicates deficiency of blood to supply the tongue; and fissures on a pale white, tender and puffy tongue with toothprints on its borders indicate invasion of dampness pathogens into deficient spleen.

Bare tongue: A bare smooth tongue of any color, like a mirror, without tongue coating is called Jingmianshe (mirror tongue), and is due to exhaustion of stomach qi; a bare tongue without a vivid appearance is caused by exhaustion of stomach Yin and depletion of stomach qi; a pale white and shiny tongue without a coating indicates damage to the spleen and stomach, and deficiency of qi and blood; and a shiny crimson tongue without a coating is due to depletion of water caused by flaming fire and exhaustion of stomach and kidney Yin.

Toothprints on the tongue: Toothprints often appear on the surrounding borders of a big and fat tongue caused by deficiency of the spleen, impairment of the metabolism of body fluids and accumulation of dampness in the body. A pale white and moist tongue with toothprints is due to accumulation of cold and dampness pathogens; and a pink tongue with toothprints is due to deficiency of spleen qi.

Double tongue: Swollen tissues and blood vessels forming a small sublingual mass is called double tongue, and the tongue is called Lianhuashe (lotus tongue) if two or three small masses appear below it, which are caused by fire pathogens in the heart due to invasion by external pathogens. This abnormal mass usually occurs in young children.

Bleeding of the tongue: Bleeding of the tongue is caused by excessive heat pathogens in the heart and disturbance of blood circulation (loss of control of blood circulation) in patients with liver fire pathogens or deficiency of the spleen.

Therefore, bleeding of the tongue is due to fire pathogens in the heart or liver, heat pathogens in the stomach, deficiency of the stomach or outward floating of Yang over the body surface.

Inflammation of the tongue: Inflammatory lesions on the tongue may invade the floor of the mouth cavity to form a red, swollen, hard and painful mass. Inflammation of the tongue is due to excessive fire and heat pathogens in the heart; and an inflammatory mass below the tongue is due to accumulation of heat pathogens in the spleen and kidneys burning off the fluids in the body.

Sore on the tongue: This is a purple bloody vesicle with an indurated painful root in the tongue proper caused by toxic fire pathogens in the heart and spleen.

Ulceration of the tongue: Painful millet-like ulcers are scattered on the borders of tongue. The bulging painful ulcers are produced by the upward gushing of toxic heat pathogens from the heart; and depressed painless ulcers on the tongue are caused by deficiency of Yin in Xiajiao (lower energizer) and upward gushing of deficient water.

Cancer of the tongue: A mass in the size of a bean on the tongue proper may gradually grow in size and assume the shape of a cauliflower or cockscomb, with a small pedicle to connect the mass to the tongue and with a red and ulcerated surface. The intake of food may be interfered with by the very painful mass in the mouth and foul saliva may constantly drip out of the mouth. This is a malignant tumor caused by accumulation of fire pathogens in the heart and spleen, stagnation of qi and upward flaming of fire. The prognosis may be better if the slowly growing tumor is not painful and ulcerated; but the prognosis is bad in patients with ulcerated tumor.

Blood vessels underneath the tongue: After the tongue is

tilted up, two bluish purple and slightly engorged blood vessels can be vaguely seen passing through the Jinjin (EX-HN 12) and Yuye (EX-HN 13) acupoints beside the frenulum of the tongue. Under normal conditions, the blood vessels are not engorged, and have no branches or petechiae. A number of bluish purple or purplish black vesicles may appear underneath the tongue, which are caused by accumulation of liver qi and blood stasis in meridians. The significance of the thick engorged blood vessels underneath the tongue is the same as that of the bluish purple tongue itself, as they are caused by accumulation of phlegm heat pathogens in the body or blood stasis due to accumulation of cold pathogens; and torsional bluish purple blood vessels are caused by stagnation of qi and blood.

4) Condition of the tongue: The condition of the tongue may be soft, stiff, tremulous, flaccid, deviated, retracted or unconsciously agitated.

Stiff tongue: The stiff tongue is rigid and inflexible, and the speech may be disturbed. There are two pathogenic causes of this: It may be caused by invasion of external heat pathogens into the pericardium to disturb the mentality and control of the tongue. The high fever may consume body fluid and cause poor nutrition of muscles and blood vessels. Therefore, the tongue loses its softness and flexibility. It may also be due to blockage of collaterals passing through the Lianquan (CV 23) acupoint caused by liver wind pathogens and phlegm; or due to upward invasion of liver Yang and wind-fire pathogens to produce poor nutrition for muscles and blood vessels, hence stiffness of the tongue. Stiff tongue indicates apoplexy (or prodromal symptoms of apoplexy) due to invasion of heat pathogens into the pericardium, exhaustion of body fluid by high fever and blockage of phlegm and turbid fluid in the body. A dark red stiff tongue proper may appear in patients with excessiveness of heat pathogens; fatty stiff tongue with thick and greasy coating may appear in patients with accumulation of phlegm and turbid fluid; and pink or bluish purple stiff tongue may appear in apoplexy patients.

Flaccid tongue: The flaccid tongue is soft and powerless to flex and protrude due to deficiency of qi and blood, and deficiency of Yin to nourish muscles and blood vessels. There are three causes of flaccid tongue: Pale flaccid tongue may appear in chronic patients with deficiency of qi and blood; dry, red and flaccid tongue may appear in acute patients with body fluid burned off by heat pathogens; and crimson flaccid tongue may appear in chronic patients with severe exhaustion of Yin.

Tremor of the tongue : Uncontrollable tremor of the tongue is caused by exhaustion of the body and wandering of wind pathogens. Tremor of the tongue may be caused by deficiency of qi and blood, depletion of Yang, exhaustion of body fluid to warm, nourish and moisten muscles and blood vessels; or be caused by wandering of wind pathogens due to severe exhaustion of body fluid by heat pathogens. The wriggling movement of the tongue in chronic patients is due to deficiency of qi and blood or deficiency of Yang; and fluttering movement of the tongue is due to wandering of wind pathogens induced by violent heat pathogens, and it may occur in patients with alcohol intoxication.

Deviation of the tongue: Deviation of the tongue to one side is due to blockage of collaterals caused by wind pathogens or wind phlegm. The deviation of the tongue to the contralateral side of paralysis of limbs is caused by apoplexy (stroke) or appears as a prodromal sign of apoplexy; purplish red deviated tongue may appear in critical patients with convulsions induced by wind pathogens in the liver; and pink deviated tongue may appear in stable patients of stroke with hemiplegia.

Playing movement of the tongue: The tongue constantly protruding out of mouth is called Tushe (protruding tongue) and repeated protrusion of the tongue from the mouth to lick the lips all around is called Nongshe (playing with the tongue). Both conditions are due to heat pathogens in the heart and spleen. The heat pathogens in the heart may induce wandering of wind, and the heat pathogens can consume body fluid to produce contraction or repeated twitching of muscles and blood vessels. Purple tongue with this symptom often appears in patients with invasion of epidemic toxic pathogens into the heart or depletion of vital energy; and it may appear in children of poor intelligence or as a prodromal sign of convulsions.

Retracted tongue: The tongue can not be protruded forward, and the retraction of the tongue is a sign of a critical disease with either a deficient or an excessive syndrome. There are four causes of retracted tongue: Pale or bluish purple, moist and retracted tongue is caused by accumulation of cold pathogens in muscles and blood vessels; fatty retracted tongue with sticky and greasy coating is due to blockage of phlegm and turbid fluid in the body; red or crimson, dry and retracted tongue is caused by wandering wind due to consumption of body fluid by excessive heat pathogens; and pale, fatty, tender and retracted tongue is due to deficiency of qi and blood.

Paralyzed tongue: The tongue protruding from the mouth can not be withdrawn and retracted into the mouth due to paralysis of the muscles of the tongue. Swollen, dry and paralyzed tongue is due to excessive heat pathogens in the muscles and attack of phlegm fire pathogens to the heart; and wide, numb and paralyzed tongue is due to deficiency of qi. Dry protruded

96

and paralyzed tongue without retractable power indicates a worse prognosis; but moist tongue with retractable power indicates a better prognosis.

(2) *Inspection of the tongue coating:*

1) Color of the tongue coating: White, yellow, grey and black are the common colors, whole green and soybean sauce colors are unusual colors of the tongue.

White coating: White thin tongue coating in normal subjects may also appear in patients with a disease caused by external pathogens still retained at the body surface; and a pale moist coating indicates an internal cold or cold and dampness syndrome. Under certain specific conditions, the white coating may indicate a heat syndrome. For example, a white chalky tongue, as if covered with a layer of wet chalk powder, indicates the invasion of external turbid pathogens and accumulation of excessive toxic heat pathogens in the body. It usually occurs in epidemic febrile diseases or in patients with bodily pain; and white coarse coating with fissures, as covered with a layer of white dry sand, indicates quick transformation and accumulation of endogenous heat pathogens and severe exhaustion of body fluid in patients of epidemic febrile diseases before the tongue coating turns yellow in color or after wrong administration of hot tonic herbs.

Yellow coating: In general, it indicates an internal heat syndrome. Light yellow coating indicates a mild heat syndrome; deep yellow coating indicates a severe heat syndrome; and roasted yellow coating indicates accumulation of heat pathogens in the body. Change of white coating to yellow color indicates the spread of external pathogens from the body surface to the interior part of the body and the transformation of exter-

97

nal pathogens to internal heat pathogens. Light yellow thin coating indicates an exterior syndrome caused by external wind-heat pathogens or due to heat pathogens transformed from wind and cold pathogens; and yellow, moist and slippery coating on a pale, fatty and tender tongue indicates deficiency of Yang and disturbance of metabolism of body fluid.

Grey coating: Grey or light black coating is transformed from dark white coating, and it may be combined with a yellow color. Grey coating indicates an interior syndrome, and it usually appears in internal heat syndrome and also in cold and dampness syndrome. Dry grey coating indicates exhaustion of body fluid by heat pathogens in febrile diseases caused by external pathogens, or indicates deficiency of Yin and excessiveness of fire pathogens in miscellaneous diseases due to injury to the internal organs; and grey moist coating indicates accumulation of phlegm and rheum or obstruction of cold and dampness pathogens in the body.

Black coating: Black coating transformed from grey or roasted yellow coating is darker than grey coating, and it indicates an interior syndrome due to violent heat or cold pathogens. It usually appears in the critical stage of epidemic febrile diseases. Black coating with fissures and prickles is caused by exhaustion of body fluid due to violent heat pathogens; and black, moist and slippery coating is due to depletion of Yang and excessiveness of cold pathogens.

Green coating and soybean sauce color coating: Green coating is derived from white coating. Same as greyish black coating, light and deep green coating always indicates a heat syndrome. Slippery and greasy coating all over the surface of the tongue with a green tint indicates transformation of Yin pathogens (cold and dampness) into heat pathogens and accu-

98

mulation of damp-heat pathogens, phlegm and rheum in patients with a damp-warm disease. The color of moldy soybean sauce is a mixture of red, black and yellow, and it is produced by transformation of turbid substance in the stomach and intestines into heat pathogens. This tongue coating may appear in patients with accumulation of heat pathogens in the body for a long time, in patients of heat stroke with stagnation of food or in patients of external febrile disease with stagnation of food and accumulation of damp-heat pathogens in the body for a long time.

2) Appearance of the tongue coating: The inspection of the appearance of the tongue coating must take into account the following: Thick or thin, moist or dry, curdy or greasy, partial or complete, exfoliated, increase or decrease and true or false.

Thick or thin coating: The criterion of thickness is whether the tongue proper is visible. If the tongue proper is faintly visible through the coating, it is a thin coating, otherwise, it is a thick coating. The thickness of the tongue coating can indicate the depth of invasion of pathogens in the body.

Thin tongue coating as a normal coating is produced by stomach qi. If the thin coating appears in patients, it indicates that the disease is not severe, the vital energy (body resistance) is not reduced and the pathogens are not very violent. Thin coating also indicates diseases caused by external pathogens or due to mild injury to internal organs.

Thick tongue coating is produced by stomach qi floating upward with turbid dampness pathogens, and it indicates the invasion of excessive pathogens into the interior part of the body, or accumulation of phlegm, rheum, dampness or food in the body.

Moist or dry coating: The normal tongue surface should be slightly moist. If the tongue surface is apparently watery in appearance, wet and slippery by palpation and saliva may drip while the tongue is protruded, it is a slippery coating; if the tongue surface is dry in appearance and by palpation, it is a dry coating; if the granules on the tongue surface look like grains of sand and give a rough sensation to the palpating finger, it is a rough coating; and it is a dry fissured coating, if the tongue surface is dry, hard and scattered with fissures. The moisture of the tongue coating can show the change of fluid in the body.

Moist coating indicates that the body fluid is not exhausted, and there is enough fluid to upwardly supply the mouth cavity. Slippery coating indicates a cold or dampness syndrome. Because Yang qi in Sanjiao (triple energizer) is deficient and the body fluid can not be metabolized in a normal manner, water in the body may be accumulated to produce phlegm and rheum, which may be upwardly transported to the mouth cavity and ooze over the tongue surface to form a slippery coating. It often appears in patients with accumulation of phlegm, rheum and dampness in the body due to deficiency of Yang.

Dryness in the mouth is due to poor supply of fluid to the mouth cavity after the exhaustion of body fluid caused by accumulation of excessive heat pathogens, deficiency of Yin, deficiency of Yang and reduced transformation of qi to upwardly transport fluid, or is caused by damage to the lungs by dryness pathogens. Dry tongue coating indicates exhaustion of fluid by excessive heat pathogens, wasting of Yin, deficiency of Yang and reduced transformation of qi to produce fluid or damage to the lungs by dryness pathogens; and a rough coating indicates wasting of fluid by excessive heat pathogens.

Under certain extraordinary conditions, a dry coating may appear in diseases caused by dampness pathogens; and the moist coating may appear in diseases caused by heat pathogens. For example, the invasion of dampness pathogens into the qi component may interfere with the transformation of qi to fluid to produce a dry coating; and the invasion of heat pathogens into the blood and the invasion of Yang pathogens into Yin may produce a moist coating, because Yin is evaporated upward by the invading heat and Yang pathogens to moisten the tongue.

Curdy or greasy coating: Coarse granules are loosely piled in a thick layer to form the curdy coating, like a layer of debris of bean curd irremovable by erasion; if the coating is dim and dirty, it is called floating dirty coating; if the tongue surface is covered with a layer of sticky and thick coating, like the pus on an ulcer, it is called purulent curdy coating; if the tongue surface is covered with a white membrane and some erosive spots in the size of grains of rice, it is called moldy curdy coating; if the fine granules are densely spread over the tongue surface, irremovable by erasing and scratching, and covered by a layer of oily mucus, it is called greasy coating; if the granules are densely glued together to form a slippery, greasy and dirty layer, it is called sticky greasy coating; and if the granules are not clearly visible and the coating is dirty and sticky, it is called dirty coating or turbid coating.

Curdy coating is produced from turbid and putrefied pathogens which can be upwardly transported from the stomach to mouth cavity in patients with excessive heat pathogens accumulated in the body, and it usually appears in patients with accumulation of food and turbid phlegm, abscess in an internal organ or oral ulceration due to damp-heat pathogens. If the firm and sticky coating can be gradually resolved and a new thin coating gradually formed, it indicates that the pathogens have been conquered by the vital energy (body resistance) and the disease will be cured; if a purulent curdy coating appears in patients with abscess of the lung, stomach or liver, or a chancre due to accumulation of toxic pathogens, it indicates a severe disease caused by violent pathogens. Moldy curdy coating is also due to putrefiction of fluid in the stomach and upward floating of turbid and putrefied pathogens.

Greasy coating is due to suppression of Yang qi and accumulation of turbid dampness pathogens in the body. It indicates a disease caused by turbid dampness, phlegm and rheum, stagnation of food, damp-heat and coagulated phlegm in the body. Yellow thick greasy coating may appear in infectious febrile diseases caused by dampness pathogens, infectious febrile diseases in summer or diseases caused by phlegm-heat and damp-heat pathogens, stagnation of food, accumulation of dampness and phlegm in the body, obstruction of hollow organs, blocking passage of qi; white slippery greasy coating may be caused by turbid dampness or cold dampness pathogens; dry thick greasy coating, like a layer of chalk powder, is caused by attack of epidemic pathogens with dampness to the internal organs of body; white moist greasy coating in patients with chest distress is due to deficiency of the spleen and excessiveness of dampness pathogens; and white, thick, sticky and greasy coating in patients with a sweet taste in the mouth is due to accumulation of damp-heat pathogens in the spleen and stomach and upward flow of accumulated qi.

Partial or complete coating: Complete tongue coating covers the whole tongue surface; partial coating covers only a localized area of the tongue surface, such as the anterior, posterior, left, right, central or peripheral area.

Complete tongue coating indicates the wide spread of pathogenss in the body and stagnation of damp phlegm in Zhongjiao (middle energizer).

Coating over the anterior area of the tongue indicates wasting of stomach qi before the invasion of external pathogens to the internal organs of the body; coating over the posterior area of the tongue indicates persistent stagnation of food in the stomach after the elimination of external pathogens; bare middle and posterior area of the tongue indicates wasting of essence, qi and blood, and reduction of upward supply of stomach Yang and kidney Yin; and coating over the middle and posterior area of the tongue indicates retained accumulation of phlegm and rheum from the past or stagnation of food in the stomach and intestines.

Coating on one side of the tongue indicates halfway invasion of pathogens to the internal organs of the body and accumulation of damp-heat pathogens in the liver and gallbladder, because the border area is the projecting region of the liver and gallbladder.

Exfoliative coating: Complete exfoliative tongue shows a tongue surface as bare as a mirror; in spotted exfoliative tongue the coating is exfoliated in spots and patches with a clear-cut margin; the new granules may appear on the tongue surface of the exfoliated area in quasi-exfoliative tongue coating.

Complete and spotted exfoliative tongue coating indicates deficiency of qi and Yin in the stomach; and spotted exfoliative tongue with a firm greasy coating around the exfoliated area indicates a complicated disease with the turbid phlegm not eliminated and the vital energy already exhausted.

Increase or decrease of tongue coating: Increase of tongue coating in area and thickness indicates increase of pathogens in the body and deterioration of disease; and the decrease of tongue coating in area and thickness indicates recovery of vital energy (body resistance) and improvement of disease. In

103

general, increase or decrease of tongue coating takes place slowly. Otherwise, it indicates a bad prognosis. For example, sudden increase of thickness of the tongue coating indicates abrupt depletion of vital energy and violent invasion of pathogens into the internal organs of the body; and sudden disappearance of a thick coating over the whole tongue indicates prompt exhaustion of stomach qi.

True and false tongue coating: True coating is firmly attached to the surface of the tongue and difficult to remove. It is called rooted coating, because the granules of the coating seemingly strike root in the tongue proper; false coating is seemingly painted on the tongue surface instead of growing from roots in the tongue proper, and it is easy to erase. Therefore, it is also called rootless tongue coating.

In the early and middle stages of a disease, rooted tongue coating indicates a more severe disease in comparison with rootless coating; but rooted coating in patients with disease in the late stage is a better phenomenon, because it indicates preservation of stomach qi in the body. If a thin layer of new coating appears underneath the original thick coating over the whole tongue surface, it indicates amelioration of disease.

For determination of false or true coating, false coating over the whole tongue surface appearing early in the morning may disappear after breakfast, and is a normal phenomenon in healthy subjects, because it is not rootless; and a tongue with a sparse coating or naked tongue after the disappearance of a false coating indicates an internal deficient syndrome. Colored coating removable by scratching indicates a mild disease; and coating removable by wiping indicates a much milder disease. If a new coating does not appear beneath a layer of rootless coating, it indicates that the original stomach qi is exhausted, and there is no more stomach qi to supply the tongue for regeneration of a new coating. This phenomenon is due to exhaustion of Yang caused by excessive administration of cold herbs or depletion of Yin after excessive administration of hot herbs.

5. Comprehensive inspection of the tongue proper and tongue coating:

In general, the tongue proper and tongue coating can be simultaneously observed because their changes are usually correspondent with each other.

(1) *Pale white tongue proper and tongue coating of various colors:*

1) Pale white tongue proper and transparent tongue coating: The tongue proper is pale white in color, and the tongue coating is white, thin and transparent as a faint true tongue coating. They indicate coldness and deficiency of the spleen and stomach, poor function of Yang in Zhongjiao (middle energizer) and upward floating of dampness and water.

2) Pale white tongue proper and white dry coating: The tongue proper is pale white in color, indicating accumulation of heat pathogens in the spleen and stomach, and deficiency of Yang and body fluid; and the tongue coating is dry, tough and coarse as sand, indicating exhaustion of the body fluid and accumulation of heat pathogens in the body.

3) Pale white tongue proper and yellow coating with fissures: A pale white tongue proper indicates deficiency of qi and fluid and upward floating of heat pathogens in weak patients; and a light yellow and fissured coating of varied thickness and moisture indicates deficiency of qi and fluid, and upward overflow of turbid dampness pathogens.

4) Pale white tongue proper and black dry coating: A pale white tongue proper and greyish black dry coating with prickles, removable by scratching, indicate excessiveness of cold pathogens in the body, deficiency of Yang and disturbance of distribution of the body fluid.

(2) *Pink tongue proper and tongue coating of various colors:*

1) Pink complete exfoliative tongue: The tongue is pink, tender, shiny and naked. This is caused by deficiency of stomach qi and Yin. This type of tongue often appears in patients with deficiency of stomach and kidney Yin or deficiency of qi and blood.

2) Pink tongue with partial white slippery coating: The white slippery coating appears merely on the left side of the pink tongue proper. It is due to wasting of Yin caused by dryness pathogens derived from damp-heat pathogens in the liver and gallbladder. Therefore, it indicates diseases caused by invasion of pathogens halfway to the internal organs of the body, diseases of the liver and gallbladder due to wasting of Yin caused by dryness pathogens or diseases due to deficiency of Yin with stagnation of dirty substance in the stomach.

3) Pink tongue with red spots and white, greasy and dry coating: This type of tongue is caused by attack of external wind-cold pathogens and accumulation of heat pathogens in the blood. Therefore, it indicates invasion of external wind-cold pathogens to the body surface, accumulation of heat pathogens in Ying (nutrient) and blood, wasting of the body fluid by excessive heat pathogens and stagnation of dampness in the spleen and stomach.

4) Pink tongue with white coating on tongue root and light

yellow coating on tongue tip: This type of tongue indicates accumulation of heat pathogens in Shangjiao (upper energizer), attack of external wind-heat pathogens to body surface and transmission of heat pathogens derived from wind-cold pathogens to the internal organs of the body.

5) Pink tongue with yellow and black coating: A yellow coarse coating covers the peripheral part of the pink tongue and a dark brown coating covers the central part of the tongue, indicating accumulation of heat pathogens with phlegm and dampness, wasting of Yin caused by dryness pathogens derived from heat pathogens and stagnation of damp-heat pathogens in the spleen and stomach.

(3) *Red and crimson tongue proper and tongue coating of various colors:*

1) Red tongue with dark, dirty and loosely attached coating: This type of tongue is caused by upward attack of dirty and turbid dampness and retained heat pathogens, and it may appear in patients with heat pathogens gradually resolved before the spleen and stomach qi are fully regenerated. Therefore, it indicates a disease caused by deficiency of vital energy and retained damp-heat pathogens not completely resolved.

2) Red tongue with white greasy coating: The tongue proper is fresh red in color with a white, moist and slippery coating, and much saliva in the mouth. If the tongue proper is tough in nature, it indicates accumulation of damp-heat pathogens in the body; and if the tongue is tender in nature, it indicates upward floating of deficient Yang and accumulation of water and dampness in the body.

3) Red tongue with black (grey) slippery coating: The tongue proper is red and fatty, and the greyish black tongue

coating mixed with white color is easily exfoliated. A bright red tongue proper indicates upward floating of deficient Yang caused by violent cold pathogens; and a slippery and easily exfoliated coating indicates a deficient cold syndrome instead of accumulation of cold and dampness pathogens in the body.

4) Red tip and borders of the tongue and a black moist coating in the central area of the tongue: The red tip and borders indicate a heat syndrome, but the central black moist coating indicates a cold syndrome in patients with a disease caused by mixed cold and heat pathogens. It appears in the following three types of disease caused by: Cold pathogens in the interior part and heat pathogens in the exterior part of the body; attack of external summer heat pathogens from outside and accumulation of cold and uncooked food in the body; and heat pathogens in the liver and gallbladder and cold pathogens in the stomach and intestines.

5) Red tongue root and black coating on the tip of the tongue: This type of tongue indicates accumulation of excessive heat pathogens in the heart.

6) Red slender tongue with black coating: A red, dry and slender tongue proper covered with a black coating indicates exhaustion of body fluid by dryness pathogens in the blood, deficiency of Yin, excessiveness of fire pathogens and wasting of fluid by excessive heat pathogens.

7) Crimson tongue with white thin coating: A dark red tongue proper covered with an uneven white thin coating (neither slippery nor dry) indicates attack of wind-cold pathogens from outside in patients with deficiency of Yin and excessiveness of fire pathogens in the past. Crimson tongue usually appears before the onset of an exterior syndrome or after the invasion of heat pathogens into Ying and blood with the

pathogens retained on the body surface not resolved. Therefore, crimson tongue is gradually formed.

8) Crimson tongue and sticky greasy coating: The crimson tongue looks dry but it is moist by palpation. Therefore, it is due to deficiency of fluid, upward evaporation of damp-heat pathogens and accumulation of turbid dampness. A crimson tongue covered with a layer of transparent, sticky and greasy substance similar to tongue coating indicates accumulation of dirty and turbid substance in Zhongjiao (middle energizer) and excessiveness of heat pathogens or deficiency of Yin, excessiveness of fire pathogens and accumulation of heat pathogens in Ying (nutrient).

9) Crimson tongue with yellowish white coating: This type of tongue indicates an invasion of pathogens from the qi component to the blood component with both components attacked by the pathogens.

10) Crimson tongue with yellow moist coating: This type of tongue is due to upward flow of water and dampness caused by heat pathogens, and it indicates the following four patterns of diseases: Diseases caused by deficiency of Yin mixed with dampness, excessiveness of fire pathogens and accumulation of damp-heat pathogens in the stomach and intestines; diseases of alcoholics caused by damp-heat pathogens in the blood and accumulation of heat pathogens in the blood component derived from dampness accumulated in the body for a long time; diseases caused by excessive damp-heat pathogens in Ying (nutrient), invasion of external heat pathogens into Ying and accumulation of more dampness than heat pathogens in the stomach and intestines; or febrile diseases caused by the external heat pathogens just transmitted from the qi to the Ying component.

11) Crimson tongue with yellow, sticky and greasy coating: A dark red tongue proper covered with a layer of yellow mucus indicates deficiency of Yin and close combination of heat pathogens in Ying with accumulated phlegm and rheum.

12) Red or crimson tongue covered with yellow coating in patches: The whole fresh or dark red tongue proper is covered with a layer of yellow, dry and thick coating, but divided into small patches, and the red color of the tongue proper can be seen in the fissures between the patches. This is caused by the coagulation of heat and dryness pathogens in the stomach and intestines and invasion of heat pathogens into Ying.

13) Red or crimson tongue with false dry coating: The tongue proper is fresh or dark red in color, and the thick or thin white coating looks dry but it is actually wet by palpation. This type of tongue is produced by two causes: The exhaustion of fluid in the body caused by damp-heat pathogens and continuous upward floating of dampness pathogens; and disturbance of distribution of the body fluid due to deficiency of qi and continuous upward oozing of dampness pathogens. A crimson tongue with thick greasy coating is due to wasting of fluid caused by damp-heat pathogens; and a pink tongue proper with false dry coating is caused by accumulation of dampness due to deficiency of qi.

(4) *Bluish purple tongue proper and tongue coating of various colors:*

1) Purple tongue with white greasy coating: A purple tongue is caused by invasion of external pathogens into the internal organs of the body to produce a thick greasy coating. This type of tongue indicates invasion of wind-cold pathogens into the body, alcoholic intoxication and excessive damp-heat pathogens

in the body.

2) Bluish purple tongue proper with yellow slippery coating: A bluish purple tongue is due to coagulation of cold pathogens and stagnation of blood in the body, and a yellow coating indicates stagnation of food, while the heat pathogens are not very excessive and the tongue coating is still moist and slippery. This type of tongue indicates coagulation of cold pathogens in blood vessels and stagnation of food in the spleen and stomach.

3) Light purple tongue proper and grey coating: A light purple tongue with grey coating, light purple tip and borders of tongue with grey coating in the central area of the tongue or a light purple color in the central area of the tongue with grey coating on the borders of the tongue are all transformed from pale white tongue proper. This type of tongue is due to wasting of blood caused by heat pathogens derived from accumulated dampness in weak patients of epidemic febrile diseases. Therefore, it indicates invasion of heat pathogens into the blood component of weak patients.

4) Blue tongue proper with yellow coating: This type of tongue may appear in patients attacked by summer heat pathogens or in patients with vomiting and diarrhea caused by invasion of cold pathogens after intake of too much cold and uncooked food. The yellow coating does not indicate a heat syndrome, because it is caused by deep invasion of cold and dampness pathogens into the blood and upward floating of heat pathogens caused by excessive Yin pathogens in the body. Therefore, it is a true cold and false heat syndrome.

5) Putaoyi tongue (epidemic disease with purpura like grapes): The tongue proper is spotted with blue or purple patches, and covered with a yellow or black coating. Blue or purple vesicles like grapes are scattered on the tongue and other

111

parts of oral cavity and the patients also suffer from sore throat, swollen lips and foul breath. This is an epidemic disease caused by accumulation of turbid, dirty and toxic heat pathogens in the body.

(5) *Critical signs of the tongue in diagnosis of diseases:*

In critical patients the tongue proper and coating may show some specific changes following the exhaustion of Yin, Yang, qi, blood and body fluid.

1) Bare tongue proper without a coating, like the kidney of a pig with the membrane peeled off: A critical sign in patients of febrile diseases with wasting of Yin or exhaustion of stomach qi.

2) Rough and dry tongue proper with prickles like fish skin: A critical sign in patients with exhaustion of body fluid.

3) Shrunken tongue proper without moisture, like a dry litchi: A critical sign in patients with exhaustion of the body fluid caused by violent heat pathogens.

4) Dark dry tongue proper with the color of pig liver or of red persimmon: A critical sign in patients with depletion of qi and blood.

5) Shortened tongue proper with retracted scrotum: A critical sign in patients with depletion of liver qi.

6) Brown tongue proper with a black tint: A critical sign in patients with depletion of kidney Yin.

7) White scales like snow flakes peeling from the tongue surface: A critical sign in patients with depletion of spleen Yang.

8) Bare tongue without coating: A sign of incurable disease due to exhaustion of stomach qi.

9) Tongue like a baked cake: A critical sign.

112

10) Bare tongue proper, like a mirror: A critical sign.

6. Inspection of the tongue and diagnosis of diseases:

According to the theory of traditional Chinese medicine, the vitality, color and shape of the tongue should be observed for diagnosis of diseases.

A pale white tongue proper, like white paper, indicates hypohemoglobinemia in patients of anemia; and a red color on both lateral borders indicates excessive fire pathogens in the liver and gallbladder in patients with fever, hypertension or hyperthyroidism.

A bluish purple tongue proper may appear in patients of chronic hepatitis, liver cirrhosis, malignant tumors, congenital heart disease, pulmonary heart disease, coronary heart disease, dysmenorrhea, irregular menstruation, endometriosis, peptic ulcer of the stomach and duodenum and chronic gastritis.

Bluish purple petechiae or spots on the tip and borders of the tongue not bluish purple in color may appear in patients with irregular menstruation, dysmenorrhea and functional uterine bleeding, or indicate blood stasis in the body. Bluish purple streaks or black spots on the bilateral borders of tongue may appear in patients of liver cancer.

Purple streaks or irregular black spots on the bilateral borders of the tongue may appear in patients of liver cancer.

The normal tongue coating is white and thin. A white thick, brownish yellow or greyish black tongue coating is seldom found in normal people, except smokers.

A white, thick and slippery tongue coating indicates accumulation of dampness in the body, and it may occur in patients with chronic bronchitis, asthma and bronchiectasis. A yellow, thick tongue coating difficult to remove even by scratching with a knife may appear in patients with superficial gastritis or relaptic peptic ulcer.

A puffy and tender tongue proper with toothprints on its borders can be clearly observed when it is protruded out of the mouth. An edematous tongue may appear in patients with malnutrition. If the tongue is permanently protruding from the mouth because it is too big to be kept in the mouth cavity, it is a specific physical sign of hypothyroidism in children. An extra-big tongue may also appear in adults with hypothyroisism or acromegaly due to hyperfunction of the pituitory gland.

Exfoliation of the coating over the central area of the tongue in patients with dryness in the mouth, reduction of secretion of saliva and pain in the tongue indicates deficiency of Yin and malnutrition; and pain in the tongue in patients with this type of tongue indicates glossitis.

Two engorged and elongated veins underneath the tongue in aged people indicate pulmonary heart disease; dilated venules like dog salmon eggs lateral to the above two veins indicate extreme senility; and a mirror tongue in aged people (especially in women) with dryness and pain in the tongue (especially remarkable after physical exertion) indicates severe deficiency of Yin.

Chapter 5
INSPECTION OF THE BODY AND SKIN, AND DIAGNOSIS OF DISEASES

Inspection of the body is an important subject discussed in this book.

I. Inspection of the Neck and Diagnosis of Diseases

In normal people, the neck is symmetrical on both sides. The neck is short and thick in short and obese people; and it is long and slender in tall and thin people. The thyroid cartilage is prominent in men; and it is flat in women. The cleidosterno-mastoid muscle may bulge when the head is turned to one side and the blood vessels of the neck are not engorged in normal people.

1. Inspection of the neck and diagnosis of diseases:

A weak neck incapable of holding up the head may appear in patients with myasthenia gracis, progressive myatrophy and chorea. Stiff neck may appear in patients of cervical spondylopathy, spasms of the cervical muscles, tetanus and diseases with meningeal irritation. Deviation of the neck may appear in patients with injury to the cervical muscles, contracture of scar, congenital trachelism (spasms of the cervical muscles) and torticollis (wryneck).

The apparent engorgement of jugular veins in standing and sitting postures indicates the increase of venous pressure in patients with right heart failure, constrictive pericarditis, pericardial effusion and superior vena cava syndrome.

Apparent pulsation of the carotid artery may appear in patients with aortic incompetence, hypertension, hyperthyroism and severe anemia.

2. Common diseases of the neck:

1) Abscess on the laryngeal prominence: This is caused by invasion of wind-heat pathogens into the lungs and stomach or by toxic fire and wind pathogens in the heart. The base of the lesion is movable. The prognosis is good, if the pus can be easily drained; but the prognosis is bad if the lesion is a hard indurated mass or the pus is drained into internal organs.

2) Abscess of cervical vertebra: This is caused by accumulation of heat pathogens in Shangjiao (upper energizer) and Dumai (governor vessel) and in severe cases the patients may suffer from spasms of the shoulder and back, nausea and vomiting. This disease with ulceration, coma and vomiting is refractory to treatment.

3) Stony mass: This is caused by accumulation of heat pathogens in the lungs, stagnation of qi and blood or accumulation of violent cold pathogens in meridians.

4) Tuberculosis of cerical lymph nodes: This is caused by attack of toxic wind, toxic heat and toxic gas pathogens. The lesions caused by toxic wind pathogens are easily ruptured, resolved and cured, and the patients may suffer from fever and chills; the slowly growing hard nodular masses caused by toxic

heat pathogens are covered with red and slightly hot skin which is seldom ruptured; and the sudden appearance of masses in the ear, neck, chest and axillary regions covered with red and hot skin are caused by toxic gas pathogens, and the patients may suffer from pain and stiffness of the neck, fever, chills, dizziness and vertigo.

II. Inspection of the Chest and Abdomen, and Diagnosis of Diseases

In normal people, the chest is symmetrical on both sides, full and round, not depressed and deviated to one side and not in a barrel shape; the ribs are slightly prominent and the intercostal spaces are not bulged; the muscles of the chest are well-developed; and the breath is even, free and regular in frequency. The abdomen is slightly bulged (on the same plane as the chest) in a standing posture, and it is slightly concave in a supine posture; the abdomen bulging over the plane of ziphoid process and pubic symphasis may appear in patients with distension of the abdomen.

1. Inspection of the chest and diagnosis of diseases:

1) Flat chest: A chest with an apparently smaller anteroposterior diameter may appear in normal thin and tall people or in patients with chronic exhaustive diseases, such as pulmonary tuberculosis.

2) Barrel chest: A chest with an equal anteroposterior and transverse diameter may appear in patients with emphysema.

3) Rickets chest: The anteroposterior diameter is increased and the transverse diameter is reduced. The lower part of the

chest is much protruded in patients with chicken chest; and the lower part of the chest is obviously depressed in patients with funnel chest.

4) Deformity of the chest: A deformed chest with local or one-sided depression, narrowed intercostal spaces, drooped shoulders and scoliotic spinal column may appear in patients with pulmonary collapse or diffuse pleural adhesion; a deformed chest with local or one-sided prominence may appear in patients with pneumothorax or marked thoracic effusion; and local protrusion of the chest may appear in patients with abscess or tumor of the chest wall.

5) Abnormal breast: Excretion of milk in unmarried women may be caused by the increased secretion of prolactin in patients with hypothyroidism and diseases of the pituitary gland or caused by disturbance of endocrinal functions in chronic thymitis, thoracic herpes zoster, chest operation and overdoses of some drugs (such as valium, metoclopramide and rifampin). Bloody discharge from the breast is a sign of malignant tumor in the breast. Hyperplasia of the mammary gland is a common disease in women with mass in the breast and local pain exacerbated before menstruation and relieved after menstruation.

2. Inspection of the abdomen and diagnosis of diseases:

In normal people, the abdomen is slightly bulged in a standing posture, and slightly concave in a recumbent posture; an abdomen bulging over the plane of ziphoid process and pubic symphasis may appear in patients with distension of the abdomen.

Physiological distension of the abdomen may appear in obese people and pregnant women.

Pathological distension of the abdomen may appear in the

118

following diseases:

Abdominal ascites: In patients with a large amount of fluid in the abdominal cavity, the abdomen may assume the shape of a frog's belly with the fluid accumulated to both flanks when lying flat; with the fluid accumulated to one side of the abdomen when lying on the side; and with the fluid accumulated in the lower abdomen in a sitting posture. Therefore, the bulging portion of the abdomen changes following the change of posture. Abdominal ascites usually appear in patients with cirrhosis of the liver, heart failure, constrictive pericarditis, metastatic cancer of the peritoneum, nephrosis and tuberculous peritonitis.

Intestinal distension: Accumulation of a large amount of gas in the intestines may produce a marked distension of whole abdomen as a ball. The flank region is not remarkably bulged and the shape of the abdomen does not change with the change of posture.

Pneumoperitoneum: Artificial pneumoperitoneum or perforation of the stomach or intestine may produce a diffuse distension of the whole abdomen.

Abdominal tumor: A large abdominal tumor, such as a huge ovarion cyst may produce a diffuse distension of the whole abdomen.

Abdominal depression: Marked depression of the abdomen may appear in patients with extreme emaciation and severe dehydration.

Localized bulging of the abdomen: Splenomegaly may cause bulging of the left upper abdomen; stomach cancer may cause bulging of the middle abdomen; and a pregnant uterus and distended urinary bladder may cause bulging of the lower abdomen.

119

Abdominal striae: Abdominal striae may appear in multipara (pregnant striae) or recovered patients of ascites or obesity. Abdominal striae may appear in patients with hyperadrenalism.

Umbilicus: The umbilicus lies at the center of the abdomen in normal subjects, and the distance between the ziphoid process and the umbilicus and that between the umbilicus and pubic symphasis are equal. Abnormal increase of the former distance indicates a lesion in the upper abdomen; and the abnormal increase of the latter distance indicates a lesion in the lower abdomen.

Abdominal body hair: In males, the body hair may extend from the sternum to the umbilicus, and the pubic hair is distributed in a triangular shape, with the tip pointed upward and extended to the umbilicus along the anterior midline of the body; in females the pubic hair is arranged in a reverse triangular shape. Abnormal increase of body hair on the abdomen or the change of distribution of pubic hair in females to the pattern of males' pubic hair indicates hypercortisolism and adrenal sexual perversion; and sparse body hair on the abdomen indicates hypofunction of the anterior lobe of the pituitary gland, myxedema and hypofunction of sexual glands.

III. Inspection of the Back and Waist, and Diagnosis of Diseases

The normal back is symmetrical on both sides and flexible in movement, and the normal physiological curvature of the spinal column can be shown in a standing posture; the waist is also symmetrical on both sides, and flexible in flexion and rotation.

1. Inspection of the back and waist, and diagnosis of diseases:

Kyphotic back with a smooth curve like the back of a turtle is due to deficiency of congenital and acquired essence, depletion of bone marrow and emptiness of Dumai (governor vessel).

Kyphotic back with an angular protrusion like the hump of a camel is due to deficiency of the kidneys, deficiency of qi and blood, poor nutrition supplied to the spinal column and injury to Dumai (governor vessel), or due to invasion of damp-heat pathogens and contracture of the spinal muscles and blood vessels for a long time.

Lordotic back with stiff neck and opisthotonus may appear in patients with tetanus and convulsions.

Rigid waist with difficulty flexing and rotating may be caused by invasion of cold and dampness pathogens, and blockage of qi in meridians, or external trauma, sprain or blood stasis in blood vessels. The pain, stiffness and difficulty of movement of the waist caused by an abscess in the region of Shenshu (BL 23) acupoint is due to deficiency of kidney qi and accumulation of cold phlegm.

Scoliosis is usually caused by the maldevelopment of the spinal column, paralysis of muscles, contracture of scar tissue and malnutrition.

Severe lumbago and difficulty walking in patients continuously groaning and turning over in bed may be caused by acute prolapse of an intervertebral disc or acute inflammation in the spinal canal.

2. Inspection of the spinal column and diagnosis of diseases:

When an internal organ is adversely affected, its projecting area on the spinal column may show an abnormal sign; for example, the T 10 vertebra may show a sensitive response to

121

pressure in patients with kidney disease (Fig. 5-1)

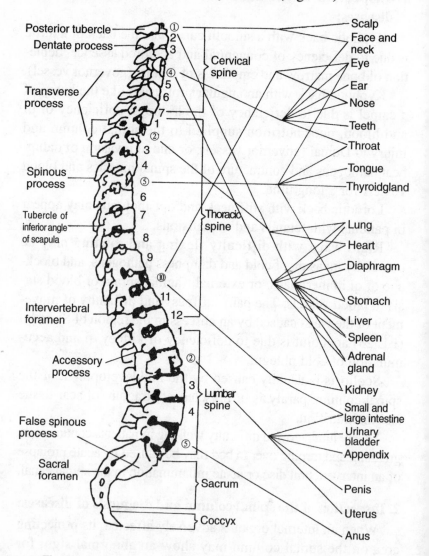

Fig. 5-1 Projecting area of organs and structures on the spinal column

The relation between the spinal nerves and their correspondent internal organs and sense organs is as follows:

(1) C 3 nerve: Diaphragm, brain, scalp, eyelid, ear, nose, mouth, teeth, thyroid gland, heart, lungs, liver, spleen, pancreas and stomach.

(2) C 4 nerve: Brain, skin of the face, eye, ear, nose, diaphragm, scalp, mouth, teeth, larynx, thyroid gland, heart, liver, spleen, pancreas and stomach.

(3) T 1 nerve: Trachea, heart, pericardium, eye, ear, diaphragm, lungs, pleura, liver and skin.

(4) T 2 nerve: Heart, trachea, ear, eye and breast.

(5) T 3 nerve: Lungs, heart, ear, eye, nose, breast, pleura, liver and skin of the body.

(6) T 4 nerve: Liver, lungs, heart, ear, breast and pleura.

(7) T 5 nerve: Stomach, eye, nose, tonsil, breast, pleura, ear and liver.

(8) T 6 nerve: Diaphragm, stomach, spleen, pancreas, liver, kidneys and breast.

(9) T 7 nerve: Diaphragm, stomach and spleen.

(10) T 8 nerve: Diaphragm, pancreas, liver, small intestine and gallbladder.

(11) T 9 nerve: Spleen, adrenal gland, pancreas, gallbladder, small intestine, stomach and diaphragm.

(12) T 10 nerve: Kidneys, small intestine, diaphragm, pancreas, spleen, gallbladder, ureter, ovaries and testis.

(13) T 11 nerve: Small intestine, diaphragm, pleura, colon, kidneys, ureter, urinary bladder, uterus, testis and ovaries.

(14) T 12 nerve: Colon, kidneys, diaphragm, peritoneum, penis, prostate gland, ovaries, testis, epididymis, uterus and spermatic cord.

(15) L 1 nerve: Urinary bladder, colon, small intestine, penis, ovary, prostate gland, uterus, spermatic cord and pleura.

(16) L 2 nerve: Appendix, penis, testis, ovaries, epididymis, spermatic cord, pleura, uterus, colon and small intestine.

(17) L 3 nerve: Penis, testis, ovaries, epididymis, urinary bladder and prostate gland.

(18) L 4 nerve: Vagina, urinary bladder, uterus, prostate gland and rectum.

(19) L 5 nerve: Prostate gland, urinary bladder and rectum.

(20) S 1 nerve: Urinary bladder.

(21) S 2 nerve: Urinary bladder.

(22) S 3 nerve: Urinary bladder, penis and vagina.

(23) S 4 nerve: Anus, penis and vagina.

IV. Inspection of Limbs and Diagnosis of Diseases

1. Inspection of limbs and diagnosis of diseases:

In normal subjects, there is an aversion angle of 5-15 degrees between the extending line of the upper arm and forearm when the elbow joint is extended. If the angle is bigger than the normal range, it is called cubitus valgus; if the angle is smaller than the normal range it is known as cubitus varus.

A flat palm without an apparent depression and with the extended thumb on a same plane as the palm indicates the paralysis of the median nerve. Difficulty putting fingers side by side indicates injury to the ulner nerve.

Continuous twitching of some muscles of the upper limb without any apparent movement of the arm may appear in patients of uremia or multiple neuritis. Tremors of the fingers may appear in patients with hyperthyroidism or neurasthenia.

Subconscious movement of the hands to seemingly grasp at something in vain or continuously rub a fixed object in chronic patients lying in bed for a long time is a critical sign of delirium caused by high fever, hepatic coma or alcoholism.

Bowleg and knock-knee may appear in rickets patients. Swollen legs with rough and thickened skin and swollen lymph nodes may appear in patients with filariasis. Enlarged knee like the knee of a crane may appear in patients of rheumatism, rheumatoid arthritis, Kaschin-Beck disease, inflammatory diseases, tumor, external trauma or tuberculosis of the knee joint.

Dizziness, blurred vision, palpitations of the heart and shortness of breath in patients with lean limbs is caused by deficiency of qi and blood. In weak people or chronic patients, weakness, leanness and tremor of the limbs, soreness and weakness of the waist and knee, and hotness in the heart, palms and soles are caused by deficiency of liver and kidney Yin; and cold body and limbs, impotence and emission of semen is due to deficiency of spleen and kidney Yang. A similar syndrome in children may be caused by deficiency of congenital and acquired kidney essence and poor nutrition of tendons, bones and muscles, and the children may also suffer from five types of retardation (of standing, walking, speaking and growing of teeth and hair) and five types of weakness (of the head, mouth, hands, feet and muscles).

Weak and flaccid limbs, lean and atrophic muscles and mental tiredness are due to deficiency and weakness of the spleen and stomach; weakness, numbness and tremor in the limbs with soreness and weakness of the waist and back, dizziness and tinnitus are due to deficiency of liver and kidney Yin.

Heaviness, weakness and numbness in the lower limbs with difficulty walking are due to paraplegia or stroke if the upper limbs are normal. Stiff limbs with difficulty flexing may appear in weak and obese people; and the stiff limbs may also be caused by deficiency of the liver and kidneys, deficiency of Yang qi or stagnation of qi and blood.

Symmetrical edema of the limbs is a local manifestation of general edema of the body. Edema of one limb may be caused by blockage of local veins or lymph vessels. Blockage of veins is caused by thrombosis of veins, paralysis of limbs or malnutrition of nerves; and blockage of lymph vessels may appear in patients of filariasis, which may cause rupture of lymph vessels, overflow of lymph, marked hyperplasia of connective tissue and thickening of skin to form elephantiasis with local non-pitting edema.

The enlarged and expanded terminals of limbs with hyper-

125

plasia of local soft tissues, bones and ligaments may appear in patients of acromegaly and giantism caused by over-secretion of growth hormone from a hyperplastic pituitary gland or acidophilic adenoma in the pituitary gland.

Muscular atrophy of the limbs may be caused by myositis, injury of peripheral nerve or disuse of muscles for a long time. Muscular spasms are due to deficiency of qi and blood and attack of wind-cold or cold dampness pathogens; and spasms of limbs with fever, chills and stiffness of the neck and back are due to blockage of meridians by wind pathogens and disturbance of circulation of qi and blood, or caused by invasion of toxic wind pathogens after trauma and disturbance of distribution of Ying (nutrient) and Wei (defensive energy).

Varicosis of the lower limbs with local redness, swelling, hotness, soreness and pain is caused by accumulation of damp-heat pathogens; varicosis of the lower limbs with swelling, heaviness, numbness, coldness and pain, exacerbated in cold cloudy weather is caused by accumulation of cold dampness pathogens; and varicosis of the lower limbs with heaviness and distension, exacerbated after tiredness, is due to deficiency of qi and stasis of blood.

Weak, drooped shoulders are due to deficiency of lung qi.

2. Inspection of the soles of the feet and diagnosis of diseases:

In traditional Chinese medicine, inspection of the soles of the feet for diagnosis of diseases is an important part of traditional diagnostics. Diseases of the internal organs can be diagnosed by observing abnormal changes in the projecting areas of those organs on the soles of the feet (Figs. 5-2 and 5-3).

When an organ in the body is diseased, some abnormal

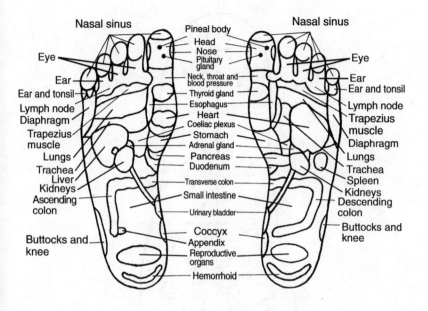

Nasal sinus   Pineal body   Nasal sinus

Fig. 5-2   Projecting areas on the soles of the feet

changes in color and shape may appear on the projecting area of that organ on the soles of the feet.

How can the diagnosis of diseases of the internal organs be made by observation of the abnormal changes of color and shape on the soles of the feet? According to the theory of traditional Chinese medicine, the meridians have their fixed origin, end points and pathways to connect different organs and structures in the body. Therefore, the pathological changes of a diseased organ can be reflectively shown on the pathway of its meridian for diagnosis of disease in the corresponding organ. According to the theory of foot reflex in Western medicine, abnormal changes on different areas of the foot can indicate

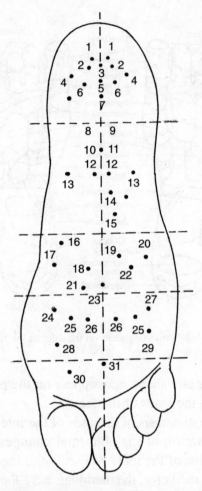

1. Brain; 2. Eye; 3. Brain stem; 4. Ear; 5. Nose; 6. Face; 7. Oral cavity; 8. Throat; 9. Thyroid gland; 10. Trachea; 11. Esophagus; 12. Bronchus; 13. Lungs; 14. Heart; 15. Cardia of the stomach; 16. Liver; 17. Gallbladder; 18. Pylorus of the stomach; 19. Stomach; 20. Spleen; 21. Duodenum; 22. Greater curvature of the stomach; 23. Pancreas; 24. Ascending colon; 25. Small intestine; 26. Kidneys; 27. Descending colon; 28. Appendix; 29. Sigmoid colon; 30. Anus; and 31. Perineum.

Fig. 5-3　Acupoints on the soles of the feet

diseases in different organs of the body (Fig. 5-4)
Fig. A and Fig. B show the relation between various areas

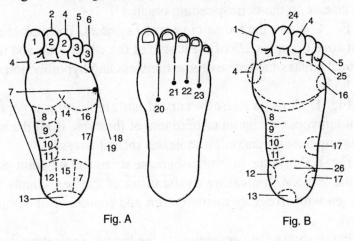

Fig. A   Fig. B

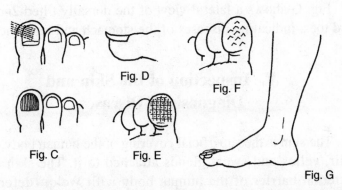

Fig. D

Fig. C   Fig. E   Fig. F   Fig. G

1. Head; 2. Hand; 3. Foot; 4. Wrist; 5. Knee; 6. Foot; 7. Gynaecology; 8. Nose; 9. Throat; 10. Chest; 11. Abdomen; 12. Lower abdomen; 13. Anus (hemorrhoid); 14. Disturbance of speech; 15. Yanggunei; 16. Back; 17. Waist; 18. Tinnitus; 19. Eye; 20. Lumbago; 21. Stomach; 22. Duodenum; 23. Gallbladder; 24. Toe; 25. Xixia (below the knee); and 26. Intestine.

Fig. 5-4   Projecting areas on the soles of the feet and diseases of different organs

on the soles of the feet and their corresponding organs. The tenderness produced by pressing the projecting area indicates the disease in the corresponding organ.

Fig. C shows the toe nail in normal subjects. The pink crescent zone occupies 1/5 of the length of the whole nail, and the vertical streaks indicate extreme tiredness and hypofunction of the body.

Fig. D shows a dorsally curved nail, indicating myopia, pseudomyopia, astigmia or tiredness of the eyes. If all the toe nails are dorsally curved, it indicates mental stress.

Fig. E shows the network of coarse striae and pinpoint pits on the big toe, indicating dysfunction of the sex glands in women with irregular menstruation and reduction of sexual desire.

Fig. F shows the unevenness of the big toe, indicating drug overdose.

Fig. G shows a lateral view of the dorsally tilted 2nd and 3rd toes, indicating diseases of the stomach and intestines.

V. Inspection of the Skin and Diagnosis of Diseases

The skin is the superficial covering of the human body, with hair, vellus and sweat glands attached to it. The skin is an external barrier of the human body with Weiqi (defensive energy) circulating through it; it is also connected with the lungs. The external pathogens first attack the skin when they invade the body; and the pathological changes of qi, blood and internal organs can also be shown on the skin through meridians.

1. Inspection of skin color:

Red skin: Fresh red skin may appear in patients with Dandu (erysipelas); the disease with red cloudy patches on the skin migrating all over the body is called Chiyou Dandu (wandering erysipelas), caused by excess of heart fire and attack of wind-heat pathogens or due to fetal poison in babies; and the local red and swollen skin on the lower limbs is called Liuhuo (erysipelas); it is due to accumulation of kidney fire and downward pouring of damp-heat pathogens.

Yellow skin: Yellow color of the skin of the body and face, eyes and nails, much deeper than the color of the skin of normal people, indicates jaundice. Bright yellow skin like orange peel in patients with yellow sweat, dark yellow urine, thirst and yellow greasy tongue coating is usually caused by damp-heat pathogens in the spleen and stomach or in the liver and gallbladder; and dark smoky yellow skin in patients with chills, tastelessness in the mouth and white greasy tongue coating is due to stagnation of cold dampness pathogens in the spleen and stomach.

Black skin: Blackish yellow skin may appear in patients with Heidan (blackish jaundice), derived from ordinary jaundice, and it is called Nulaodan (sexual intemperance jaundice) if caused by sexual intemperance. Dark black or blackish sallow skin of face or whole body at the late stage of edema is due to extreme exhaustion of kidney essence. Black or brown patches on the skin are caused by stagnation of liver qi and blood stasis, accumulation of damp-heat pathogens in the body, deficiency of Yin and excess of fire pathogens, or deficiency and dysfunction of the spleen.

2. Inspection of the moisture of the skin:

Moist skin and hair indicate sufficiency of Taiyin qi; dry

skin and hair indicate deficiency of Taiyin qi; shrunken skin and loss of hair indicate lung damage; and dry haggard skin and broken hair indicate exhaustion of lung Yin. Inspection of the hair and vellus can determine the nature of a disease (deficient, excessive, cold or heat) and the location of pathogens (superficial or deep). Erect hair and vellus is due to attack of deficient pathogens in patients with chills. In general, dry and broken vellus indicates a bad prognosis; and moist and intact vellus indicates a good prognosis.

Skin as dry as fish scales is known as Jifu Jiacuo (dry scaly skin), and the patients with this type of skin and dark eyelids may suffer from abscess or accumulation of dry blood in the body if they also suffer from acute pain in abdomen.

Lichenous skin like snake slough all over the body and ulcerated skin without pus are all signs of Lifeng Pibing (skin lesion of leprosy).

3. Inspection of swelling and distension of the skin:

Swelling of the skin (edema) may appear on the head, face, chest, abdomen, back, waist and limbs; and distension (ascites) appears only on the abdomen. Diseases in patients with swollen supraclavicular fossa, soles of the feet, back and umbilicus due to edema are difficult to cure.

In patients with thin and bright skin, local or general edema is often pitting in nature. Edema starting from the face and spreading to the limbs and rest of the body in patients with symptoms of common cold is called Fengshui (edema caused by wind pathogens) due to impairment of dispersion of lung qi and blockage of circulation of body fluid; edema starting from the limbs and slowly spreading to the rest of the body in patients with tiredness of limbs, poor appetite and diarrhea is due to accumulation of water and dampness in the spleen and dysfunction of the spleen; and edema starting from the waist and lower limbs and gradually spreading to the rest of the body, but more remarkable in the waist and lower limbs of patients with soreness and weakness of the waist and knee, coldness in the stomach, cold limbs and clear urine is due to deficiency of kidney Yang and impairment of the metabolism of the water in the body.

Dim, lusterless and swollen skin without pitting is due to stagnation of liver qi and poor circulation of qi; and local red swollen skin with intractable itching and pain is due to insect bite or caused by insect poison accumulated in the skin and muscles.

4. Inspection of poxes on skin:

Pealike poxes on skin are often accompanied with symptoms of exterior syndrome. The pox lesions of the skin can be divided into smallpox and chicken pox ones.

Smallpox: Round poxes of different sizes may appear simultaneously with red halo, deep root, depressed vesicle pit and turbid vesicular fluid like pus, and the pock marks may be retained on the face after the crusts have been peeled off.

Chicken pox: Oval poxes of different sizes may appear in succession with thin vesicle membrane easily ruptured, clear thin vesicular fluid but without vesicle pit, thick crust and pock marks left on the face.

5. Inspection of skin rashes:

Skin rashes contain macules and papules. The red, flat and smooth macules not detectable by palpation can be divided into Yin and Yang types; and the red miliary papules detectable by palpation may appear in measles, German measles and urticaria.

Yin macules: The Yin macules vary from coin to pinpoint in size and from pink to deep purple in color, indistinct in appearance, less in number and indeterminate in location, but they are invisible on the head, face and back. The patients are mentally clear and have cool limbs and thready and weak pulse.

Yang macules: This skin lesion is caused by invasion of warm pathogens of infectious febrile diseases into Ying (nutrient) and blood, accumulation of heat pathogens in the lungs and stomach, widespread heat pathogens all over the body and transmission of excessive heat pathogens from Ying and blood to superficial skin and muscles. The macules are produced by heat pathogens in the muscles; and the papules are caused by heat pathogens in blood vessels.

A few red macules and papules may appear on the chest and abdomen first, spread to the limbs with fever, and then disappear after reduction of the fever, and they indicate a good prognosis of a mild disease with pathogens all eliminated; but dense deep red or purplish black macules and papules may appear on the limbs first, and then spread to the chest and abdomen with persistent high fever and coma, and they indicate a critical disease caused by invasion of pathogenss into internal organs when the pathogenss are dominant over the body's resistance. Dull, black and haggard skin rashes indicate a critical disease. Diseases in patients with papules are mild; but diseases in patients with macules are severe. Red sparse skin rashes indicate a mild disease; but dense dark red skin rashes indicate a severe disease, and dim black rashes indicate a critical disease.

Measles: This is an common infectious disease of children. Before the onset of the disease, the patient may suffer from cough, sneezing, running nose with clear discharge, brimming tears in the eyes, cold ears and red streaks behind the ears; 3-4 days later, sparse, pink, pointed and sesame-like papules palpable by the hand may appear and spread from the head and face to the chest, abdomen and limbs, with the skin rashes gradually increasing in number. The prognosis is good in children with slight sweating, full eruption and gradual resolution of bright red skin rashes and fever gradually subsiding; but the prognosis is bad in children with high fever, coma, asthma and incomplete eruption or sudden subsidence of dull pink rashes (attack of wind cold pathogens to the body surface), dark reddish purple rashes (excessive toxic heat pathogens in the body) or pale pink rashes (deficiency of vital energy) on the skin without sweating because the disease is caused by inward invasion of toxic pathogens of measles.

German measles: This is a common infectious disease caused by wind heat pathogens. The skin lesions are small, pink, sparse and slightly bulged vesicles with intermittent itching and low fever. The daily life and work of patients is not disturbed by this disease.

Urticaria: Large patches of confluent papules, pale pink in color and bulging over the surrounding skin may be produced by scratching due to deficiency of Ying and blood, and attack of wind pathogens into meridians, disturbing the blood circulation. Skin rashes may appear and disappear from time to time; they are therefore called hidden papules.

6. Inspection of crystalline sudamina and vesicles:

Crystalline sudamina and vesicles are prominent blisters on the skin. The crystalline sudamina are the small papular vesicles and the vesicles are the blisters of different sizes. Crystalline sudamina are the small white prominent granules like millet grains on the skin. If the blisters are as shiny as crystal, the disease is mild; the disease is severe if dim, shrunken blisters due to exhaustion of qi and Yin are present for a long time; and the disease is critical if the blisters are dry and white like dead bone in appearance due to depletion of qi and blood and loss of vital energy from the body after elimination of pathogens. Crystalline sudamina may repeatedly recur in damp-warm infectious diseases with damp-heat pathogens retained in the body.

Herpes simplex is clusters of blisters from pinpoint to mung bean in size distributed on the borders of the lips near the mouth angle, eyelids, prepuce and external genital organs, with an itching and burning sensation. Herpes simplex usually appears in normal subjects or patients with high fever caused by stagnation of wind-heat pathogens in the lungs and stomach, and attack of heat pathogens to the skin.

Prickly heat is the dense red granular lesions with pointed tips, itching sensation and pricking pain. It usually appears in children and obese people in the summer due to accumulation of damp-heat pathogens in the skin and muscles.

Eczema produces multiform skin lesions. Early erythematous lesions may gradually swell to form papules and vesicles, then red and moist erosive skin lesions with exudate are formed after the blisters are ruptured, and finally some scars are left after the dry crusts of the healed lesions have been peeled off. This skin disease is due to accumulation of wind, dampness and heat pathogens in the skin and muscles or deficiency of blood to nourish the skin and muscles; and in chronic patients it is due to wasting of blood, and production of endogenous wind and dryness pathogens in the body.

7. Itching of the skin and diagnosis of diseases:

Itching of the skin is a common symptom of skin diseases, and it may be a preliminary sign of liver diseases, or lymphocytic reticuloma or other tumors. The itching may be divided into general and local types. General itching of the whole body is related to temperature, season, environment, food, pregnancy, allergy to drugs and many general diseases, including diabetes mellitus, liver diseases, kidney diseases and disturbance of the endocrinal system. In local itching, itching of the scrotum is related to poor local hygiene or deficiency of vitamin C; itching of the anal region is related to pinworm, proctitis and perineal eczema; and perineal itching in women may be caused by leukorrhagia, vaginitis, pregnancy, infection of the urinary tract, gonorrhea, liver diseases, kidney diseases and diabetes mellitus.

8. Skin as a mirror of bodily health:

Extremely pale skin indicates anemia while red skin indicates high RBC count and high susceptibility to diseases of the heart, liver and intestine. In patients with avitaminosis A, the skin is dry, desquamated, susceptible to pyogenic infection and covered with cornified hair follicles; in deficiency of riboflavin, the patient may suffer from seborrheic dermatitis, scrotitis, angular stomatitis and glossitis; in avitaminosis C, the cutaneous blood vessels are fragile, resulting in subcutaneous bleeding by trauma.

VI. Inspection of the Perineal Region and Diagnosis of Diseases

The perineal organs contain the anus and external genital organs of men and women.

Swollen scrotum without itching or pain may be caused by sitting on damp ground or by attack of wind, and it may be a manifestation of severe general edema; transparent swollen scrotum is called Shuishan (water hernia), and is due to accumulation of water; and opaque soft swollen scrotum is called Hushan (fox hernia), and is due to prolapse of the intestines. Swelling and pain of the testes is also included in Shan (diseases of the genital organs), and it can be divided into qi, blood, Jin (penis), swelling, cold, water and fox types caused by stagnation of liver qi, attack of cold pathogens, accumulation of damp-heat pathogens, deficiency of qi or standing for a long time. Swelling of the vaginal orifice without pain is due to local edema; and swelling of the vaginal orifice with pain is due to damage of blood component by overfatigue.

Inward retraction of the penis, scrotum and orifice of the vagina is due to stagnation of cold pathogens in meridians or invasion of external heat pathogens into Jueyin meridian to cause depletion of Yin fluid and poor nourishment of external genital organs. Red, itching and painful ulceration of the penis with purulent discharge is caused by damp-heat pathogens in the liver. The normal scrotum in healthy children with sufficient qi is firmly contracted and purplish red in color; but it is loose, suspended and white in color in weak children with deficiency of qi and blood.

Prolapse of the uterus from the vagina is called Yinting or Yinqie in traditional Chinese medicine, and it is due to deficiency of Zhongqi (qi in the middle energizer) and descent of spleen qi, or is caused by delivery injury or damage produced by extraordinarily heavy physical work after childbirth. White, dry and haggard skin with severe itching in the perineal region of women is called valvar leukoplakia, and is due to dysfunc-

138

tion of the liver, spleen and kidneys or disturbed circulation of qi and blood through Chongmai (thoroughfare vessel), Renmai (conceptional vessel) and Dumai (governor vessel).

Ulcerated external genital organs with bloody or purulent discharge are due to syphilis or unhealthy sexual activity.

Sparse pubic hair in women may appear in the following diseases: Hypothyroidism with gradual loss of pubic, axillary and scalp hair, reduction of sexual desire, fear of cold, constipation, sleepiness, general weakness and amenorrhea; dysfunction of the pituitary gland with loss of scalp and pubic hair, pathological leanness, reduction of sexual desire and amenorrhea after profuse uterine bleeding during childbirth; and Turner's syndrome with sparse pubic hair, dwarfism, underdevelopment of the breasts, delayed menarche, oligomenorrhea or amenorrhea.

VII. Inspection of Posture, Gait and Gesture and Diagnosis of Diseases

1. Inspection of posture and diagnosis of diseases:

Abnormal postures are useful for the diagnosis of diseases.

Active posture: Active posture without limitation of movement may appear in patients with mild diseases.

Passive posture: The posture of the body and the position of the limbs can not be actively changed in extremely weak or unconscious patients.

Forced supine posture: Patients with acute peritonitis are constrained to take a supine posture with both legs flexed to reduce the spasms of the abdominal muscles.

Forced prone posture: Prone posture can reduce spasms of

the back muscles in patients with diseases of the spinal column.

Forced lying on the side: Patients with pleuritis or marked pleural effusion prefer to lie on the diseased side to reduce their suffering.

Forced sitting posture: Patients with poor heart and lung function prefer to sit on a chair with the hands placed on the knees or on the chair to support the body, improve the breathing, decrease the return of blood to the heart and reduce the burden on the heart.

Forced squatting posture: Patients with congenital cyanotic heart diseases are often constrained to squat down or take a knee-chest position to release their sufferings of shortness of breath and palpitations of the heart when they are walking.

Forced standing posture: Patients with angina pectoris are often constrained to stop walking and to stand still with their hand pressing the precordial region for relief from sudden attack of precordial pain.

Turning over posture: Patients with gall stone or biliary ascariasis may repeatedly turn over in bed and feel uneasy when standing or sitting during the sudden onset of severe abdominal pain.

2. Inspection of gait and diagnosis of diseases:

The gait is the manner of walking.

Reeling gait means the body sways alternately to both sides (duck gait), and it may appear in patients with rickets, Kaschin-Beck disease, progressive myodystrophy and congenital dislocation of the hip joint.

Drunken gait is an unsteady and incoherent way of walking, as seen in drunken men, and it may appear in patients with cerebellar diseases, alcoholism or barbital poisoning.

Ataxic gait may appear in patients with tabes dorsalis, walking with the foot raised high and put down suddenly, and with the eyes looking downward to carefully watch the road. The feet are placed far away from each other to maintain an erect posture, and the balance of the body can not be maintained when the eyes are closed.

Festinating gait may appear in patients with Parkinson's disease, walking with small and quick steps, and with the body inclined forward, seemingly difficult to stop walking.

Stepping gait may appear in patients with paralysis of the common peroneal nerve with foot drop and flaccid muscles, and the tendons around the ankle joint are loose. Patients have to walk with their lower limbs raised high. In addition, patients with deformity or injury of the lower limbs or diseases of the joints may display other different abnormalities in walking.

3. Inspection of gesture and behavior, and diagnosis of diseases:

Gesture and behavior are motions and conditions of the human body. The trunk is upright and regular, and the movement of the limbs is nimble and flexible in normal subjects. But the movement of the neck is limited in patients with cervical diseases; the body is doubled up in patients with abdominal pain; and patients with gastric and duodenal peptic ulcer or colic pain in the stomach and intestines often hold their stomachs with their hands when they walk.

Muscular twitching of the eyelids, face, lips and fingers (toes) is a sign of the approach of convulsions in febrile diseases caused by external pathogens; and it indicates the stirring up of endogenous wind in miscellaneous diseases due to injury to the internal organs.

141

Convulsions or spasms of the limbs with stiffness of the neck and back and opisthotonus may appear in patients with epilepsy, tetanus, hydrophobia or convulsions due to production of endogenous wind from violent heat pathogens and stirring up of liver wind; and tremor of the head, body and limbs, with the hands making subconscious movements indicates deficiency of vital energy and stirring up of liver wind.

Bodily shaking may appear in malaria before sweating or diseases with struggle between pathogens and vital energy (body resistance); subconscious movement of the hands to grasp the air or to rub the clothes or blanket indicates a critical disease with unconsciousness.

Weakness and immobility of limbs without pain is Wei-syndrome (paralysis), and is due to deficiency of the liver and kidneys; swollen and aching joints with limitation of movement is Bi-syndrome; and disuse, numbness, contracture or flaccidity of limbs is due to paralysis of the muscles.

Sudden onset of coma, hemiplegia and deviation of the mouth and eyes are caused by attack of wind to the solid internal organs; violent convulsions in acute patients are caused by excessive heat pathogens; mild convulsions in chronic patients are caused by deficient wind pathogens; sudden coma with smooth breath indicates Jue-syndrome (syncope); sudden coma with opened mouth, relaxed hands and incontinence of urine is a stroke (apoplexy) of the open type; sudden coma with locked jaw and clenched fists is a stroke of the closed type; sudden coma in summer with flushed face and sweating is a summer stroke; and patients with flexed body and immovable waist supported by the hands are suffering from pain in the waist and leg.

If the patient is curled up under a heavy overcoat, it indicates an external or internal cold syndrome; if the patient is averse to heat and wants to undress, it indicates an external or internal heat syndrome; if the patient buries his or her head to avoid light, it indicates eye disease; if the patient holds his or her head high to watch bright objects, it indicates a heat syndrome; patients with Yang syndrome prefer coldness and wish to have companions; patients with Yin syndrome prefer warmth and wish to be alone; patients with Yang, heat and excessive syndrome may suffer from annoyance and like to stretch out their limbs, talk endlessly and constantly move the body, but are averse to heat; and patients with Yin, cold and deficient syndrome may suffer from heaviness of the body and difficulty turning over in bed; they like to curl up, put on a heavy coat and remain silent.

Patients with deficiency of lung qi prefer to sit with the body curled up; patients with adverse qi in excessive lungs prefer to sit with the limbs stretched out; orthopnea (shortness of breath while lying down) may be caused by distension of the lungs with cough and asthma or be due to accumulation of water and rheum in the chest and abdomen; tiredness and vertigo in patients restrained in bed may be caused by deficiency or exhaustion of qi and blood; patients with preference for standing up over sitting down may suffer from diseases caused by water, phlegm and rheum; and patients with annoyance and restlessness may suffer from distension and pain in the abdomen.

Patients with Yang, heat and excessive syndrome can freely turn over in bed and prefer to lie with the face exposed to the light and the legs extended; and patients with deficiency of Yang and averse to cold tend to lie in bed with the body curled up.

Chapter 6
INSPECTION OF THE HAND AND DIAGNOSIS OF DISEASES

The normal palm is clean, bright, moist, depressed in the central area and prominent in the peripheral area; the thenar and hypothenar prominences bulge; the fingers are full and flexible; the dorsum of the hand is thick with full interosseous spaces and unexposed metacarpal bones except the metacarpophalangeal joints; the veins on the dorsum of the hand are not engorged or distorted; the fingers gradually and slightly narrow toward the tips of the fingers, and they can keep close contact with each other without apparent gaps between them; the creases of the palm and fingers are continuous and symmetrical; the finger nails are convex, smooth and shiny rectangular plates occupying 3/5 of the distal phalanxes, and the distal free edge of the nail is wider than its proximal border; normal nails are symmetrical, without deviation, deformity, vertical or horizontal fissures or interference spots; and the crescent located along the proximal border of the nail is not opaque.

The grasping power of males is 20-45 kg; 5-40 kg in females.

The normal hand is bright reddish yellow in color. The temperature of the dorsum is same as that of the skin of body and it is higher in palm of hand.

I. Inspection of the Nails and Diagnosis of Diseases

The nails can show the condition of the internal organs, including the heart, liver, spleen, lungs and kidneys.

The color and crescent of the nail should be carefully observed for diagnosis of diseases, and the presence of a proper crescent on each nail indicates a good general health. The normal crescent occupies 1/5 of the nail in area, and the absence of a crescent or the presence of only a trace of a crescent indicates tiredness or sickness.

The nails are varied in shape, and can be divided into regular, large, small, long, short, wide and narrow types.

1. Inspection of the shape of the nails and diagnosis of diseases:

Thin and fragile nails indicate chronic wasting diseases, such as anemia and disturbance of the endocrine system; large, thick and hard nails with vertical fissures indicate stagnation of liver qi, with annoyance, anger, distension of the chest and flank, dizziness and bitter taste in the mouth; nails with bilateral edges ingrown into the soft tissue indicate insomnia and hysteria.

Clubbed finger: The tip of the finger is expanded like a pestle, with a bulging nail caused by intoxication or prolonged insufficient supply of oxygen to the extremities, as seen in patients of emphysema, lung cancer, congenital heart disease, cirrhosis of the liver, malignant tumor or ulcerative colitis. It may also appear in patients with hereditary defects or poor nutrition from childhood.

Tuberculous nail: The nails in patients of tuberculosis may

145

be large and round, like a clam shell or a spoon.

Arcuate nail: The nails bulge along the midline and are depressed on both edges like a bow; this condition may appear in patients of arteriosclerosis or cancer.

Fusiform finger: The interphalangeal joints are expanded like a spindle; this condition may appear in patients of rheumatoid arthritis.

Flat nail: Flat nails may appear in patients with indigestion or chronic gastritis.

Deformed nail plate: Depressed grooves or thimble-shaped pits on the nail may appear in patients with dryness in the mouth and throat, soreness and weakness of the waist and knee, sweating during sleep and palpitations of the heart due to deficiency of Yin, excessiveness of fire and dryness pathogens in the blood and muscles.

Soft nail: Soft and fragile nails may appear in patients with diseases of the spinal column and spinal cord.

Big nail: Slender fingers with big nails occupying 1/2 of the distal phalanx in area may appear in patients susceptible to diseases of the respiratory system.

Horizontal threads on the nails are a prodromal sign of critical cardiac infarct; horizontal grooves on the nails may appear in weak patients with chronic wasting diseases; fine pits on the nails indicate drug intoxication, nicotine intoxication in smokers or parasites in the body; white flocculent spots on the nails indicate neurasthenia, the yellow spots on the nails indicate digestive diseases, and blackish yellow spots indicate kidney diseases or extreme weakness. Fissures like chive leaves along the nail grooves indicate parasites in the body.

The nails are also related to the beats of the heart and pulpation of blood vessels; abnormal pulsation of capillaries underneath the nails indicates aortic incompetence or congenital patency of the arterial duct. Abnormal pulsation can be clearly seen while gently pressing the free edge of the nail.

2. Inspection of nail color and diagnosis of diseases:

The nails of healthy subjects are light pink in color; pale white nails indicate anemia or long-term malnutrition; yellow or yellowish green and slowly growing nails without crescents may appear in patients with chronic bronchitis, icteric hepatitis or psoriasis; blue nails are due to administration of certain drugs; purplish black and cynotic nails are due to pulmonary heart disease and severe hypoxia in the brain tissues; brown and opaque nails are caused by fungus infection; greyish black nails or nails with black stripes are due to increase of melanin in patients with hypoadrenalism; yellowish black nails are due to increase of hemosiderin; and nails with vertical brown fissures or white flocculent spots may appear in patients with diseases of the intestinal tract.

II. Inspection of the Fingers and Diagnosis of Diseases

1. Inspection of the blood vessels on the thenar prominence and diagnosis of diseases:

The thenar prominence is a lump of muscles through which the lung meridian passes. Blue blood vessels on this prominence indicate cold pathogens in the stomach; red blood vessels indicate heat pathogens in the stomach; the sudden appearance of black vessels indicates Bi-syndrome; a mixture of red, black and blue vessels indicates attack of mixed cold and heat pathogens; and blue short blood vessels indicate deficiency of qi.

2. Inspection of different parts of the fingers and diagnosis of diseases:

The relationship between the hand and internal organs is shown in Fig. 6-1.

(1) *Thumb:*

The thumb corresponds to the respiratory organs.

Thick clubbed thumb indicates congenital heart disease or bronchiectasis; and a slender distal phalanx of thumb covered with shrunken skin indicates prolapse of the rectum, incontinence of urine and ptosis of internal organs due to deficiency of qi.

(2) *Index finger:*

The index finger corresponds to the heart, liver, pancreas, head, stomach and intestines. Stiff index finger may appear in people with a very good appetite or a hot temperament due to excessive fire pathogens in the liver.

(3) *Middle finger:*

It corresponds to the heart and kidneys.

(4) *Ring finger:*

It corresponds to the nervous system. Inflexible ring finger may appear in patients with epilepsy or deafness.

(5) *Little finger:*

It represents the kidneys and the reproductive organs. Slender distal phalanx of the little finger indicates deficiency of kidney qi.

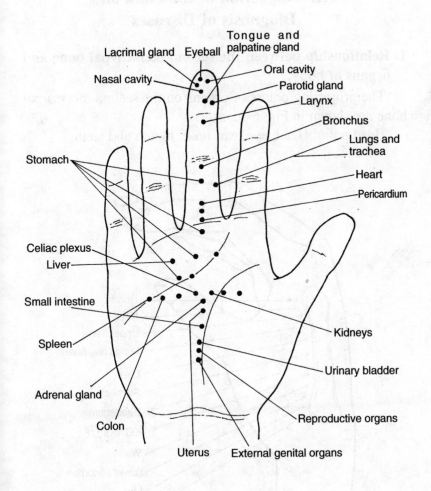

Fig. 6-1   Relation between the hand and internal organs

149

III. Inspection of the Palm and Diagnosis of Diseases

1. Relationship between the second metacarpal bone and organs of body:

The projecting points of organs on the second metacarpal bone are shown in Fig. 6-2.

Head point: Head, eye, ear, nose, mouth and teeth.

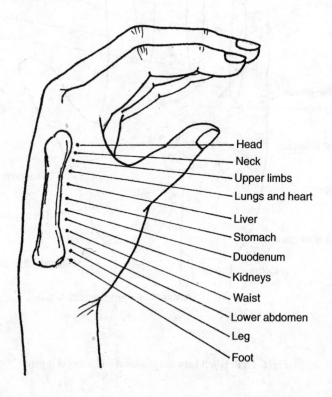

Fig. 6-2   Projecting points of organs on the second metacarpal bone

Neck point: Neck, pharynx, larynx, thyroid gland, upper segment of the trachea and esophagus.

Upper limb point: Shoulder, elbow, hand, wrist, upper limbs, middle segment of trachea and esophagus.

Lungs and heart point: Lungs, heart, chest, breast, back, bronchus, lower segment of the trachea and esophagus.

Liver point: Liver and gallbladder.

Stomach point: Stomach, spleen and pancreas.

Duodenum point: Duodenum and colon.

Kidney point: Kidneys, umbilical region, colon and small intestine.

Waist point: Waist, colon and small intestine.

Lower abdomen point: Lower abdomen, uterus, urinary bladder, rectum, appendix, ovaries, vagina, testis, urethra and anus.

Leg point: Leg and knee.

Foot point: Foot and ankle joint.

Usage of projecting points on the second metacarpal bone for diagnosis of diseases: The tip of the thumb of the examiner is used to knead and press 12 projecting points in succession with an even pressure, once or several times. A sore, numb, distending and heavy sensation at any projecting point produced by the kneading and pressing manipulation indicates a disease in the organ corresponding to that point.

2. Inspection of the color of the palm and diagnosis of diseases:

The palm of a healthy subject is pink in color. Dark red palm indicates poor heart function; the sudden appearance of black tea color on the palm is a prodromal sign of cerebral hemorrhage; yellow or sallow palm indicates liver disease; yellow palm with congestive bloody red color or dark purple patches on the tips of the fingers or thenar and hypothenar prominences indicates cirrhosis of the liver or liver cancer; blue palm with apathic facial expression indicates anemia or kidney disease; engorged blue blood vessels on the dorsum of the hand indicate accumulation of feces in the intestines; sallow palm in patients with a dark forehead indicates dysfunction of the stomach and intestines, with abdominal distension and belching; light yellow, dry and lusterless palm indicates deficiency of spleen and stomach qi, and deficiency of qi and blood; and bluish yellow palm indicates stomachache caused by cold pathogens in the stomach.

3. Inspection of sweating of the hand and diagnosis of diseases:

Constant sweating from the palms of patients with a hot sensation in the palms and soles of the feet is due to deficiency of blood; cold sweating from the palms of patients with cold hands and feet indicates deficiency of qi or Yang; sweating from one palm only indicates blockage of qi and blood in meridians; continuous oozing of sweat from the palms in patients with extremely cold limbs indicates collapse due to depletion of qi and Yang; and sweating from the palms in patients with fever not reducible is caused by endogenous heat pathogens in the body.

IV. Inspection of the Shape of the Hand and Diagnosis of Diseases

1. Inspection of the shape of the hand and diagnosis of diseases:

Claw hand: Semiflexed hand seemingly holding something

is due to paralysis of the muscles of the hand caused by injury to the spinal nerve roots in patients with progressive myoatrophy, ischemic muscular contracture of the forearm or leprosy.

Monkey hand: Similar to the palm of a monkey, with muscular atrophy of the thenar prominence and failure of the thumb to abduct in patients with paralysis of the median nerve, progressive myoatrophy, carpal tunnel syndrome and poliomyelitis.

Fan-shaped hand: As a specific sign of acromegaly, the hand is as thick and broad as a fan, with many deep creases on the skin. The fingers are thick and short, with round and enlarged terminals and big square nails.

Spade hand: The fingers are short and puffy, the soft tissue is edematous, the skin of the fingers is pale, dry, rough, loose and cold, but the skin on the dorsum of the hand is tough and shrunken, and the nails are short and broad, with ridges and in a spoon shape. This is typical of patients with myxedema.

Sclerodermatous hand: The short, slender, hard and semiflexed fingers can not be fully extended, the pads of the fingers disappear, and the nails are curved and thickened. This is typical of patients with scleroderma.

Mongolism hand: The little finger is short and concaved to the ring finger, and the second segment of the little finger is particularly short. It may appear in patients of mongolism with dementia facial expression, wide distance between the eyes and tongue protruding from the mouth cavity.

2. Projecting areas on the hand indicating common diseases:

The projecting areas on the hand indicating common diseases are shown in Fig. 6-3.

Darkness and dryness on a projecting area of the hand indicates dysfunction or disease of its corresponding organ.

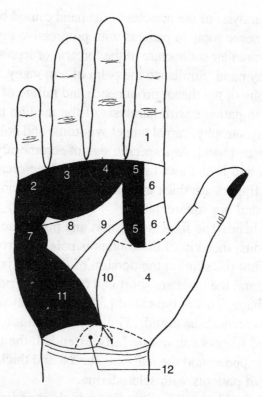

1. Gallbladder; 2. Reproductive organs; 3. Visual organs; 4. Heart; 5. Stomach; 6. Liver; 7. Kidneys; 8. Blood pressure; 9. Nervous system; 10. Digestive system; 11. Circulatory system; and 12. Reproductive organs and kidneys.

Fig. 6-3 Projecting areas on the hand indicating common diseases

Blue color, darkness and dryness in the liver area and white color and dullness in the stomach area indicates cirrhosis of the liver, liver cancer or late stage of hepatitis.

Red color in the heart area with an irregular border indicates acute attack of rheumatic myocarditis, acute infectious endocarditis and viral myocarditis; and white color in the heart area indicates ischemia of the heart muscles.

Red color in the stomach and gallbladder areas indicates chronic gastritis, stomach hemorrhage or early stage of cholecystitis; black ring in the stomach area indicates formation of ulcer in the stomach; and black color and dryness in the stomach area indicates vertigo and tinnitus due to deficiency of vital energy.

White color over a large part of the digestive system area indicates prolapse of the rectum, chronic diarrhea or ptosis of the stomach due to deficiency of Zhongqi (qi of the middle energizer).

Darkness over the whole palm indicates general diseases due to impairment of immunity.

3. Inspection of prominences of the hand and diagnosis of diseases:

People in ancient times named the prominences of the hand after the sun, moon and stars (Fig. 6-4).

The prominences of healthy subjects are pink in color, slightly bulging and elastic.

Dark red color over the Mars and moon prominences indicates apoplexy (stroke); greyish black color on the Jupiter prominence indicates dysfunction of stomach and intestine; dark spots on the Venus prominence, along the life line and between the Jupiter and first Mars prominence indicate liver diseases; and the change of the above dark spot to a dark red color indicates cirrhosis of the liver; dark or greyish black streaks between Jupiter and Saturn prominence indicate severe dysfunction of the digestive system; red spots near the above streaks indicate acute digestive diseases; the color of a withered leaf in the central area of the sun prominence is a critical sign, and

155

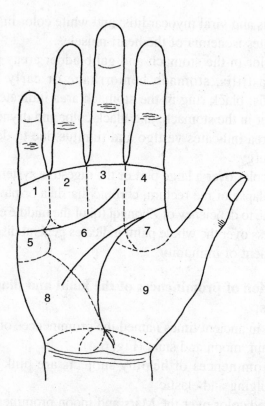

1. Mercury prominence; 2. Sun prominence; 3. Saturn prominence; 4. Jupiter prominence; 5. Second Mars prominence; 6. Plain of Mars prominence; 7. First Mars prominence; 8. Moon prominence; and 9. Venus prominence.

Fig. 6-4   Prominences of the hand

the risk of disease is in proportion to the size of the abnormal color; checked or crisscross lines in the lower area of the moon prominence indicate urinary diseases; black color, dryness and dullness on the moon prominence indicate diseases of the kidneys; and abnormal depression or red patch in the ulnar area of the moon prominence indicates critical heart disease or cerebral hemorrhage.

4. Inspection of the creases of the hand and diagnosis of diseases:

There are many creases on the palm, but the life line, love line, wisdom line and health line are the most important (Fig. 6-5).

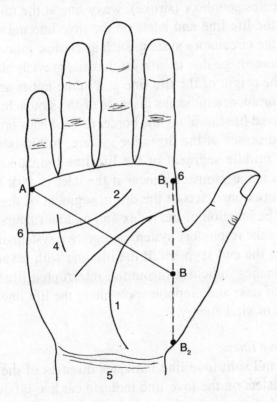

1. Life line; 2. Love line; 3. Wisdom line; 4. Health line; 5. Wrist line; 6. Origin.

Fig. 6-5 Creases of the palm

157

In normal subjects there are three continuous wrist lines. Wrist lines convexed to the palm side in women indicate infertility, abortion or difficult labor; and discontinuous wrist lines indicate diseases of the reproductive organs.

(1) *Life line*:

The sudden disappearance of the distal segment of the life line indicates apoplexy (stroke); wavy line at the middle segment of the life line and islets on the love line indicates diseases of the circulatory system, such as cardiac infarct and cerebral hemorrhage due to arteriosclerosis; greyish black color around the origin of the life line and in the upper area of the Venus prominence indicates diseases of the stomach; islets on the concaved life line along the border of the Venus prominence indicate diseases of the digestive system; turbid islets at the upper or middle segment of the life line indicate a serious disease, such as stomach cancer if the islet is dark brown in color; continuous islets at the origin segment of the life line distal to the junction of the index and middle fingers indicate diseases of the respiratory system or digestive system; deep grey color over the end segment of the life line with several crisscross branches indicates insomnia; interrupted life line is a warning of risk; and pinpoint spots along the life line indicate reduction of vital energy.

(2) *Love line*:

Dark and split love line indicates diseases of the ear and kidneys; islets on the love line indicate cardiac infarct; islets on the love line proximal to the ring finger indicate cataracts or glaucoma; a normal love line should stop at the extended midline of the middle finger through the palm, and a love line shorter than this normal standard indicates diseases of the circulatory system.

(3) *Wisdom line*:

The interruption of the wisdom line indicates dysfunction of the brain and nervous system; the normal wisdom line should stop at the extended midline of the ring finger, and a wisdom line shorter than this normal standard indicates rhinitis or otitis media; people with chainlike wisdom line across the whole palm may often suffer from headaches; sudden stoppage of the wisdom line at the midline of both palms indicates functional disturbance of the brain; intersection of the life line with the terminal segment of the wisdom line indicates mental depression; interruption and splitting of the wisdom line is a prodromal sign of neurosthenia; and abnormal wisdom line and love line indicate hysteria.

(4) *Health line*:

The health line originates from a point proximal to the junction of the ring and little fingers, and obliquely passes along the border of the moon prominence toward the life line. Abnormal color over a short health line indicates diseases of the digestive system; interrupted health line indicates diseases of the digestive system; islets on the segment of the health line near the life line indicate severe diseases of the digestive system; red or black spots along the health line are a prodromal sign of fever; a curved snake-like health line indicates damage to the liver caused by alcoholism; an interrupted fine health line in women indicates gynaecological diseases caused by cold pathogens; bigger islets on the health line indicate diseases of the respiratory system; a fine black health line passing across the life line indicates heart diseases; and red color at the inter-section of the health and love lines indicates susceptibility to heart diseases.

Chapter 7
INSPECTION OF EXCRETA AND SECRETA, AND DIAGNOSIS OF DISEASES

The excreta are waste products of the metabolism discharged from the body, and the secreta are secretions discharged from the sensory organs. The inspection of stool, urine, sputum, slobber, nasal discharge, spittle, blood, sweat, pus, vomitus, menstrual blood and leukorrhea for diagnosis of diseases is discussed in this chapter.

I. Inspection of Stool and Urine, and Diagnosis of Diseases

The stool and urine are important metabolic products discharged from the body through a series of complicated metabolic processes. The change of amount and nature of stool and urine can not only show the state of health and presence of diseases of the digestive and urinary systems, but it also reveal the condition of many other organs.

1. Inspection of stool and diagnosis of diseases:

The normal stool is passed once a day or every two days with a proper consistence and a banana shape, but it does not contain blood, pus, mucus or undigested food.

The increase of quantity and times (more than two times a day) of defecation indicates indigestion or enteritis; the discharge of dry and hard stool is called constipation; the discharge of watery, loose and unformed stool is known as diarrhea; flat tapelike stool is caused by constricture of the anus or rectum cancer; undigested food in loose stool is a sign of diarrhea due to deficiency of the spleen or kidneys; and white pus in stool indicates dysentery.

The normal stool is yellow or brown in color and the abnormal stool may be green, greyish white, red or black in color. Green stool is due to salmonellal food poisoning or intake of too much vegetable; greyish white stool is due to obstructive jaundice; fresh red stool containing blood in the feces is due to bleeding of the anus or rectum in patients with anal fissure, hemorrhoids, rectal polyps or rectal cancer; dark yellow stool is due to hemolytic jaundice; blackish red or tarry stool indicates bleeding of the upper digestive tract; shiny stool mixed with many fat droplets is due to intake of too much fat in the food or poor digestion of fat in patients with diseases of the pancreas; stool in the color of fish brain indicates dysentery caused by damp-heat pathogens; and blue stool is due to invasion of wind pathogens into the stomach and intestines.

The urgent sense of defecation in patients without stool passed out is known as tenesmus in patients of dysentery; dry stool with a granular appearance is due to accumulation of heat pathogens in the colon; difficulty passing a formed stool is due to deficiency of the spleen and lung qi; and the incontinence of stool is due to deficiency of spleen and kidney qi or descent of deficient qi.

The normal stool is a pastry column in shape. Stool like goat feces indicates constipation; flat tapelike stool is due to constricture of the anus; watery stool with mucus, pus or blood is due to acute gastroenteritis; stool with mucus and blood is due to amoebic dysentery; and stool with pus and blood is due to acute bacterial dysentery.

2. Inspection of stool of infants and diagnosis of diseases:

The meconium (feces of a newborn baby) is dark green, sticky and odorless, and it may turn yellow in color 2-3 days after the meconium is all evacuated. Stool of breast-fed infants is a golden yellow homogeneous paste with a sour smell; but the stool of infants fed with cow's milk is a light yellow muddy plaster with a foul smell.

Watery stool of infants is due to indigestion, infantile diarrhea or enteritis; stool like bean dregs is due to fungal enteritis; dark brown, watery and foamy stool with a sour smell is due to intake of food rich in starch; stool with fresh blood attached to its surface or its terminal segment is due to bleeding from anal fissure or rectal polyps; dark red pasty stool or watery stool like red bean soup is due to necrosis of the intestines with bleeding; and tarry stool indicates bleeding of the stomach or duodenum.

Besides bleeding of the digestive tract, black stool may also be caused by swallowing of blood in a large amount from the nasal or oral cavity, intake of pig's liver or animal blood, or administration of iron preparation for anemic patients; and the stool may turn red in color after administration of rifampin, which may cause a misdiagnosis of hemorrhage of the digestive tract.

Stool of infants mixed with mucus like nasal discharge may appear in patients with colitis or chronic bacterial dysentery; and stool of infants mixed with pus, blood and mucus is often

163

due to bacterial dysentery; clay-colored stool is due to blockage of the biliary tract without bile discharged into the intestines; and fatty diarrhea in infants with a large amount of light yellow watery or pasty stool with a bad smell is due to intake of too much fat in the food or dysfunction of the pancreas.

3. Inspection of urine and diagnosis of diseases:

In normal adults the discharge of urine in 24 hours is about 1,000-1,500 ml, and the amount of urine discharged in a day accounts for two-thirds or three-fourths of the total quantity of liquid in a day. The amount of urine is related to the intake of water, nature of food, sweating and the weather.

If the daily amount of urine is less than 500 ml, it is called oliguria; it is called auria if the daily amount is less than 100 ml. Pathological oliguria may appear in patients with severe vomiting, diarrhea, burn injury over a large area of the body surface, high fever, shock or acute nephritis; and pathological auria may appear in patients with acute renal failure or severe toxic shock. If the daily amount of urine is more than 2,500 ml, it is called polyuria, and pathological polyuria may appear in patients with diabetes mellitus, diabetes insipidus or chronic nephritis.

The uncontrollable discharge of urine is called incontinence of urine, and true incontinence of urine may appear in patients with infection, stone in the urinary tract, tuberculosis or tumor of the urinary bladder or urethra due to persistent increase of muscular tension of the pubovesical muscle in the urinary bladder or due to over-relaxation of the sphincter muscles of the urethra; and congenital incontinence of urine may appear in patients with congenital deformity of the urinary tract.

164

Normal urine is a light yellow transparent liquid, but the color of urine may change to yellow, red, brown, green, blue or white after intake of some drugs or food. The color of urine can provide information for diagnosis of diseases. Light yellow urine may appear in normal subjects after drinking much water or in patients of diabetes insipidus, polyuria or diabetes mellitus; deep yellow urine may appear in normal subjects after drinking less water or after profuse sweating or in patients with damp-heat pathogens in the liver; dark yellow urine like concentrated tea may appear in patients of acute hepatitis with jaundice or obstruction of the biliary tract; brown urine like soy sauce may appear in patients of favism with hemolysis in the blood vessels and hemoglobinuria; white urine may appear in patients of filariasis with chyluria or in patients of purulent infection of the urinary tract with pus in the urine; white turbid urine may also appear in normal subjects with a large amount of crystals of salts in the urine while drinking less water in the cold season; dark green or blue urine may appear in patients of cholera and typhus or after intravenous injection of methylene blue dye; and brownish black urine may appear in patients of paroxysmal myoglobinuria after physical exertion.

Bloody urine is called hematuria, and it can be caused by injury to any part of the urinary tract, including acute nephritis and stone, tuberculosis or tumor in the urinary tract. Hematuria can be divided into the microscopic type, with RBC visible only under the microscope, and the gross type, with apparent bloody urine visible with the naked eye. Hematuria may appear in patients with blood diseases or infectious diseases; dark red urine may also occur after a severe crush injury to the body, with hematoporphyrin in the blood and urine; and red urine may appear in normal subjects after intake of red dye.

II. Inspection of Sputum, Slobber, Nasal Discharge and Spittle, and Diagnosis of Diseases

Sputum is turbid and sticky excreta from the lungs and trachea, and the clear thin discharge from the respiratory tract is called rheum; mucous fluid can also be excreted from the nasal cavity; slobber is a clear, thin and mucous fluid dripping from the mouth; and spittle is a foamy mucous fluid spat from the mouth.

1. Inspection of sputum and diagnosis of diseases:

Sputum must be fresh for observation by the naked eye to make a diagnosis of diseases.

Mucous sputum: Colorless or pale white transparent mucous sputum may be discharged by patients of acute bronchitis and early stage of pneumonia if the amount of the sputum is not much; sputum is sticky, foamy and white in color in patients of chronic bronchitis; and sputum is scanty and sticky in patients of viral pneumonia or allergic pneumonia.

Serous sputum: In patients of bronchiectasis without apparent infection the sputum is thin, transparent, foamy and easy to spit out in a large amount; and in patients with pulmonary edema sputum is a bloody and foamy serous discharge.

Purulent serous sputum: A large amount of sputum is collected in the morning and stored in a glass jar, and then it can be divided into three layers. The upper layer contains the purulent foam, the middle layer is a thin serous fluid and the lower layer is composed of turbid, purulent and necrotic debris. Purulent serous sputum, sometimes with a foul smell, is usually spat out by patients of bronchiectasis with infection or lung abscess.

Purulent sputum: A large amount of yellow or yellowish green sputum mixed with sticky coagula or opaque purulent fluid amounting to several hundred ml per day may be spat out by the patients of lung abscess, bronchiectasis with infection, pulmonary tuberculosis with cavity or late stage of lung cancer with infection.

Bloody sputum: Bloody streaks and clots in sputum or mouthfuls of fresh blood may be spat out by patients of pulmonary tuberculosis and bronchiectasis; rusty sputum may be spat out by patients of lobar pneumonia; dark red sputum may be spat out by patients of pulmonary infarction; orange red or brownish red sputum like peach jam may be spat out by patients of paragonimiasis; and sputum with bloody streaks may be spat out by patients of lung cancer.

According to the theory of traditional Chinese medicine, yellow sticky sputum with coagula is produced by heat pathogens; white thin sputum with greyish black particles is produced by cold pathogens; clear, thin and foamy sputum is produced by wind pathogens; white slippery sputum in large amounts and easy to spit out is produced by dampness pathogens; scanty sticky sputum difficult to spit out is produced by dryness pathogens; fresh blood in sputum is due to damage to the blood vessels of the lungs by heat pathogens; and the spitting of foamy rheum by patients with shortness of breath through mouth is due to atelectasis of the lungs.

Rusty sputum is caused by destruction of red blood cells in sputum to release hemosiderin in patients of lobar pneumonia.

Shitan (food sputum) is a large amount of sticky sputum like peach jam or clam meat; Jiutan (alcohol sputum) is a large amount of sticky sputum spat out and with nausea; and Qitan (qi sputum) is accumulated in the throat to produce a sensation of a foreign body.

Healthy people do not spit out any sputum or only spit some

mucous fluid.

2. Inspection of slobber and diagnosis of diseases:

Slobber is a mucous fluid dripping from the corner of the mouth. This is due to heat pathogens in the stomach or parasites in the intestines; and white sticky slobber is due to deficiency of the spleen and accumulation of damp-heat pathogens. Slobber in infants is a normal phenomenon, because they are still very young and the reflex of swallowing saliva has not been established. Increase of saliva may appear in children with heat pathogens in the stomach or with glossitis, gingivitis or ulcers in the oral cavity; and increase of slobber may appear in children with dementia or cretinism due to disturbance of the mental, nervous or endocrinal functions, and the patients may also suffer from poor intelligence and other symptoms of endocrine diseases.

Dripping of slobber, deviation of the mouth and eyes and hemiplegia often appear in adult patients of apoplexy due to deficiency of spleen qi to control the overflow of saliva.

3. Inspection of nasal discharge and diagnosis of diseases:

A small amount of nasal discharge is constantly excreted in normal people to moisten the nasal cavity and clear away dust, but it is a pathological symptom if a large amount of nasal excretion is constantly discharged.

Turbid nasal discharge is due to attack of external wind-heat pathogens; clear nasal discharge is due to attack of external wind-cold pathogens; constant excretion of turbid nasal discharge is a symptom of rhinitis; excretion of clear nasal discharge with nasal obstruction is due to attack of wind-cold pathogens to the lungs; excretion of nasal discharge with fever and coughing indicates a common cold; and excretion of nasal discharge, coughing, sneezing, sighing, annoyance, swollen face and red cheeks are the prodromal signs of measles.

The excretion of watery nasal discharge may appear as a prodromal sign of some infectious diseases (such as measles and scarlet fever) or occur in patients of allergic rhinitis, acute rhinitis, influenza, common cold caused by wind-cold pathogens, and trigeminal neuralgia; sticky purulent nasal discharge may be excreted by patients of chronic rhinitis, lupus of the nose and chronic paranasal sinusitis; nasal discharge like bean dregs may be excreted by patients of caseous rhinitis; extraordinary foul nasal discharge may be excreted from patients with chronic atrophic rhinitis or foreign body in the nose; and nasal discharge with bloody streaks may be excreted from patients with external trauma or cancer of the nose.

4. Inspection of spittle and diagnosis of diseases:

The ejection of a large amount of spittle is caused by accumulation of food, or of cold or dampness pathogens in the stomach, or may be due to deficiency of the kidneys and accumulation of cold pathogens in the kidneys. In normal people the daily discharge of saliva is about 1,000-1,500 ml, and it is a pathological phenomenon if the amount of saliva is too large or too small.

III. Inspection of Sweat, Pus and Vomitus, and Diagnosis of Diseases

1. Inspection of sweat and diagnosis of diseases:

The sweat is a product of body fluid excreted from body

surface after evaporation of body fluid by Yang qi in body to moist the skin and adjust body temperature. The abnormal sweating in patients can show the sufficiency of Yang qi and body fluid and the struggle between pathogens and vital energy (body resistance).

The color of sweat may be yellow, red or black.

The yellow sweat may stain the clothes into yellow color and it is due to attack of external damp-heat pathogen to skin and muscles; and the yellow sweat may appear in patients of jaundice with yellow urine, yellow eyes, yellow tongue coating, bitter taste in mouth and stringy, slippery and rapid pulse.

The red sweat, also called bloody sweat may stain the clothes into red color.

The sticky sweat usually appears over the head of patients with deficiency of kidney qi and Yin and it may quickly turn black in color and continuously perspire right after the sweat on skin is wiped off; the foul sweat may be perspired from patients with acute rheumatic arthritis or acute exacerbation of chronic rheumatic arthritis; and the persistant perspiration of turbid foul sweat after subsidence of fever in patients of febrile diseases is due to accumulation of dampness, turbid fluid and residual heat pathogen in body.

2. Inspection of location and nature of sweating and diagnosis of diseases:

Spontaneous sweating: The spontaneous sweating is due to disturbance of Ying (nutrient) and Wei (defensive energy) or deficiency of qi and Yang while it is not caused by physical exertion, hot weather, putting on heavy overcoat or administration of antipyretic.

Sleep sweating: The sweat is perspired during sleep and it

stops after waking up. It is due to deficiency of Yin and the body fluid is evaporated out of body by endogenous deficient heat pathogen.

Profuse sweating: The profuse sweating within a short interval can be divided into excessive and deficient types. The profuse sweating with fever, thirst and desire to drink cold water may appear in patients of febrile diseases at the crisis stage; and the profuse sweating with cold limbs, weakness of body and shortness of breath may appear in patients with deficiency and damage of internal organs due to deficiency of Yang and failure to retain the body fluid in body.

Exhaustion sweating: The profuse and dripping sweating in critical patients with cold skin is a fetal sign due to exhaustion of Yang.

Sweating with chillness: The perspiration after chillness in patients of febrile diseases due to attack of external pathogens is a manifestation of struggle between pathogens and vital energy (body resistance). If the body is cool and the pulse is moderate the prognosis is good because the pathogens are under control; but the prognosis is bad if the high fever is persistent and the pulse is still rapid because of the deterioration of disease.

No sweating: The absence of sweating in patients with a disease which ought to cause sweating is due to attack of excessive wind-cold pathogen to body surface and retention of cold and dampness pathogens in body surface.

Sweating over head and face: The sweating limited to the head and face is a normal phenomenon in babies during sleep or in adults having a meal; the pathological sweating over head and face in raining season is caused by the attack of mixed dampness and internal heat pathogen and the upward evaporation of damp-heat pathogen in patients with fever, weakness of body, scantiness of urine and jaundice; and the aged people with poor conserving energy due to deficiency of Yang may have cool sweat on head and face, pale complexion, cold limbs and deep and thready pulse.

Sweating on nose: The patients with severe pain in heart and spleen due to deficiency of Yang and accumulation of cold pathogen in body may have cool droplets of sweat on nose bulb.

Sweating over precordial and chest region: It can be divided into qi deficiency and Yin deficiency types. In qi deficiency type, the sweating over precordial and chest region is due to damage of heart and spleen qi, deficiency of Yang qi in chest, discharge of body fluid from body caused by worriment, improper diet (too hungry or too full) or physical tiredness in patients with palpitation of heart, shortness of breath and poor appetite; and in Yin deficiency type, it is caused by sexual indulgence, wasting of kidney essence, stirring up of deficient heat pathogen in body and external discharge of heart Yin in patients with deficiency of Yin, annoyance and hot sensation in heart, palms and soles.

Fishy smell sweat: The sweat of patients with liver cirrhosis is light yellow in color and fishy in smell.

Fragrant sweat: The sweat of patients with diabetes malletus may produce an aromatic smell.

Deficient sweating: In patients of hyperthyroidism with enhanced metabolism and increased production of heat, the deficient sweat is discharged to adjust body temperature and release heat from body.

Axillary sweating: It can be divided into damp-heat type and Yin deficiency type. The meridians of liver and gallbladder pass through the axillary pit. In damp-heat type, the sweating from axillae is caused by damp-heat pathogen accumulated in liver and gallbladder, disharmony of liver collaterals and disturbance of sweating; and in Yin deficiency type, it is due to deficiency of liver Yin and blood and forced perspiration by endogenous heat pathogen.

Sweating over waist: The sweating over waist without apparent cause is due to deficiency of kidney qi.

Sweating from scrotum: The discharge of cool sweat is due to deficiency of kidney Yang and the discharge of sticky sweat is due to downward pouring of damp-heat pathogen.

Sweating of hand and foot: The hands and feet receive qi supplied from stomach and spleen and the constant sweating on hand and foot through four seasons is due to evaporation of fluid by heat pathogen from spleen and stomach to four limbs. It may be accompanied with sleep sweating of whole body.

Sweating on one half of body: The sweating of left, right, upper or lower one half of body may be due to disturbance of Ying (nutrient) and Wei (defensive energy) and poor conservation of qi and blood in patients with sallow complexion, tiredness and weakness; or caused by conjugation of wind pathogen and phlegm and stirring up of wind pathogen in meridians of patients with dizziness and tremor of hands and feet as a prodromal sign of stroke.

2. Inspection of pus and diagnosis of diseases:

The pus is the putrefied fluid in skin and muscles. The thick pus indicates the preservation of enough vital energy in body, but the thin pus indicates the deficiency of vital energy. The increase of thickness of pus indicates increase of vital energy and amelioration of disease, and the decrease of thickness of pus indicates the decrease of vital energy and deterioration of disease.

The pus in a bright color indicates a better prognosis than that in a dark color. The bright light yellow thick pus indicates the sufficiency of qi and blood; the bright light yellow thin pus indicates enough conservation of vital energy; the yellow, turbid and thick pus indicates a benign pathological process although the pathogens have not been eliminated; the blackish green thin pus indicates the inward invasion of toxic pathogen to attack tendons and bones; the pus mixed with purple blood clots indicates the damage of blood vessels; the yellow pus like ginger juice in patients with jaundice indicates a critical disease; the fish-smelled pus without foul odor indicates a benign pathological process; and the fishy and foul pus indicates a malignant pathological process.

3. Inspection of vomitus and diagnosis of diseases:

The contents of vomitus expelled from stomach are varied, including food, clear water, sputum, rheum, pus and blood and the nature, color and amount of vomitus can reveal the causes of vomiting.

The cold vomiting of thin vomitus without foul smell is caused by impairment of digestion, stagnation of water in stomach and impairment of downward transporting function of stomach due to deficiency of spleen and kidney Yang or attack of cold pathogen to stomach; and the hot vomiting of thin, turbid, sour and foul vomitus is caused by upward overflowing of heat pathogen from stomach after the attack of heat pathogen to stomach or due to accumulation of fire pathogen in liver.

The vomiting of indigested food with sour and foul smell due to food stagnation is caused by injury of spleen and stomach after overeating, stagnation and prolonged putrefication of

174

food and inhibition of downward transportation of stomach qi; and the vomiting of indigested food without sour and putrefied smell due to qi stagnation is caused by reverse overflowing of stagnated liver qi.

The vomiting of clear watery phlegm and rheum in patients with chest distress and greasy tongue coating is due to impairment of spleen function, stagnation of fluid in stomach and upward regurgitation of phlegm, rheum and stomach qi; the vomiting of yellowish green bitter fluid is due to accumulation of warm or heat pathogen in liver and gallbladder, adverse attack of liver qi to stomach, impairment of downward transporting function of stomach and forced regurgitation of bile by heat pathogen.

The vomiting of fresh blood or dark purple blood clots mixed with food fragments is due to accumulation of heat pathogen in stomach, attack of liver fire to stomach or disturbance of blood circulation to cause bleeding and accumulation of blood clots; and the vomiting of a mixture of blood and pus is due to abscess in stomach.

The vomiting of indigested food is due to indigestion; the vomiting in patients with diarrhea is due to food intoxication or acute gastroenteritis; the vomiting in patients with abdominal pain and constipation is due to intestinal obstruction; and the projectile vomiting may appear in patients of epidemic meningitis or encephalitis B.

IV. Inspection of Menstrual Blood and Leukorrhea, and Diagnosis of Diseases

1. Inspection of menstrual blood and diagnosis of diseases:
The menstrual blood is discharged for 3-5 days once a

month and the normal menstral discharge is red in color and proper in amount. The abnormal cycle, amount, color and nature of menstrual blood is defined as disturbance of menstruation.

(1) *Vaginal bleeding:*

The vaginal bleeding is a gynaecological disease different from normal menstrual flow, including profuse, prolonged and irregular menstrual discharge and contact bleeding. The causes of vaginal bleeding are varied in patients at different age: The vaginal bleeding in young girls or menopausal women may be caused by organic lesions; in women at adolescent stage it may be caused by functional uterine bleeding; and it may be related to pregnancy in women of childbearing age.

(2) *Color of menstural discharge:*

The dark red sticky menstrual blood in a large amount and mixed with clots is due to heat pathogen in blood; the pink thin discharge is due to deficiency of qi; the dark vaginal discharge with clots is due to blood stasis; the amount and color of menstrual flow may be constantly changed in patients with stagnation of liver qi; the foul vaginal discharge indicates a heat syndrome; and the fishy smell of vaginal discharge indicates a cold syndrome.

(3) *Dysmenorrhea:*

Dysmenorrhea is a gynaecological disease with abdominal pain or other discomforts before, during and/or after menstrual period.

Primary dysmenorrhea: The dysmenorrhea of this type may be caused by nervous tension, depression, frightening, emotional disturbance, anemia or other chronic diseases, spasm of

176

cervix, stenosis of cervical orifice or canal, severe declination of uterus and dysplasia of uterus.

Secondary dysmenorrhea: The dysmenorrhea of this type may be caused by contraction of uterine muscle, local congestion and stenosis of cervical canal in patients with polyps or myoma in uterus, endomytriosis and pelvic infection, including inflammation of oviduct or ovary, pelvic peritonitis and cellutitis.

(4) *Amenorrhea:*

The amenorrhea can be divided into the primary, secondary and physiological types.

Primary amenorrhea: It appears in girls without menarche after 18 years of age due to diseases of reproductive organs or pituitary gland, severe malnutrition in adolescent stage or severe tuberculosis. Besides amenorrhea, the adolescent patients with congenital hyperplasia or tumor of adrenal cortex may also suffer from symptoms of virilism, such as acne, protrusion of thyroid cartilage and enlargement of clitoris.

Secondary amenorrhea: The regular menstrual cycle may be stopped over three months in patients with diseases of uterus, ovary or thalamus due to mental stress or malnutrition.

Physiological amenorrhea: It may appear in women of pregnancy, breast-feeding or menopause as a normal physiological phenomenon.

False amenorrhea: The amenorrhea of this type is due to imperforate hymen and stenosis of vagina or cervical canal.

In traditional Chinese medicine the diseases of menstruation can be divided into Benglou (profuse vaginal bleeding), Elu (drippling vaginal bleeding) and irregular menstruation.

Benglou: The profuse vaginal bleeding may be caused by

177

failure of liver to store blood and failure of spleen to control blood circulation due to damage of liver by fury and attack of spleen by liver, or due to damage of uterus by sexual coitus in menstrual period.

Elu: The pink scanty vaginal blood may be continuously discharged by drops for several days in weak patients with qi deficient to conserve blood; and the drippling of dark blood is often accompanied with abdominal pain.

Irregular menstruation: The menstrual flow may be markedly disturbed, either antedated or postponed, either profuse or scanty and abnormal in color. It is caused by overfatigue, attack of external wind-cold pathogen, sexual indulgence or poor menstrual hygiene.

2. Inspection of leukorrhea and diagnosis of diseases:

The normal leukorrheal discharge is a white thin fluid excreted from vagina without blood and bad smell, but the nature and amount of the vaginal discharge may be markedly changed in patients with leukorrheal diseases.

Color of leukorrhea: The normal leukorrhea is a white clear discharge, but the yellow or yellowish green is an abnormal color of leukorrhea. The leukorrhea in red, brown and black color is stained by the blood in patients with tumor of oviduct, endometrium or cervix; and the greyish leukorrhea with blood streaks may be discharged from patients with vaginal ulcer, pyogenic vaginitis, cervicitis or foreign body in vagina.

Amount of leukorrhea: The moderate amount of leukorrhea may be discharged from women in ovulation stage or by the strong stimulation of estrogen and mental stress; and the profuse discharge of leukorrhea may appear in patients with vaginal ulcer, pyogenic vaginitis, cervicitis, foreign body in vagina and tumors of reproductive organs.

Nature of leukorrhea: The mucous leukorrhea is discharged in ovulation stage or by strong stimulation of estrogen and mental stress; the foamy leukorrhea is discharged in trichomonal vaginitis; the leukorrhea like bean dregs is discharged in fungal vaginitis; and the watery leukorrhea is discharged from patients of vaginitis, cervicitis or tumor of endometrium and oviduct.

Accompanied symptoms of leukorrhagia: The abnormal leukorrhea with itching of external genitalia may be discharged from patients of trichomonal vaginitis and fungal vaginitis; the abnormal leukorrhea with vaginal bleeding is discharged from patients of endometrial infection, polyps of cervix and carcinoma of cervix or uterine body; and the abnormal leukorrhea with abdominal pain may be discharged from patients of myoma of uterus or carcinoma of uterine body.

The foul and mouldy leukorrhea may be discharged from patients of trichomonal vaginitis, cervicitis and tumor of cervix, endometrium or oviduct.

Chapter 8
SELF-DIAGNOSIS OF BODILY HEALTH
AND DISEASES

I. Self-diagnosis of Diseases by Pulse Diagnosis

1. Self-diagnosis of diseases by pulse diagnosis:

The pulsation of arteries is palpated with the fingers for diagnosis of diseases of patients or the examiners themselves. As mentioned in the *Yellow Emperor's Internal Classic* (an ancient medical classical work): "A good physician can determine the Yin or Yang nature of diseases by observing the facial complexion and palpating the pulse."

In ancient times, there were three methods of pulse diagnosis: General palpation, palpation at the three arteries and palpation at the radial artery; but at the present time, only the last method is practised. The pulsation at the radial artery can be divided into 28 patterns according to depth, frequency, shape and tendency, to diagnose diseases in the human body.

The radial artery is divided into three portions, the Cun, Guan and Chi segments. The Guan segment is medial to the radial capitulum, the Cun segment is distal to it and the Chi segment is proximal to it. The palpation may be applied at three levels of depth, the superficial, and intermediate and deep levels. The palpation of pulsation at three portions of the artery and at three levels of depth can obtain 3x3=9 items of information of pulse diagnosis. The Cun, Guan and Chi segments of the left hand are the projecting portions of the heart, liver and kidneys; and the three segments of the right hand are the projecting portions of the lungs, stomach and Mingmen (life gate).

The palpation of the radial artery medial to the radial capitulum is an important method of diagnosis to find the nature of the pulsation of arteries, the changes of qi and blood, the sufficiency of Yin and Yang, and the etiology, nature and prognosis of diseases.

Palpation of the artery by the fingers uses three different pressures: the touching, moderately searching and pressing methods. As mentioned in *Essentials of Diagnosis* written by Hua Boren: "The gentle palpation is to just touch the artery; the heavy palpation is to forcibly press the artery; and the intermediate palpation is to moderately press the artery and ascertain its property." The general palpation at three portions of the artery by three fingers and the localized palpation at one portion by a single finger should be combined to perform a complete pulse diagnosis. The index finger is used to palpate the Cun segment of the artery with the middle and ring fingers, not touching the artery, and in the same manner the middle finger and ring finger are used to palpate the Guan and Chi segments of the artery, respectively.

Pulse diagnosis is better performed in the early morning. The examiner should maintain a natural and even breath as when performing pulse diagnosis and the breath of the examiner is used to count the frequency of pulsation. The duration of palpation for pulse diagnosis should be longer than 50 beats of pulsation.

The pulse can be divided into the normal and diseased types.

The normal pulse of healthy subjects should be rich in stomach qi and vitality, with a solid foundation. The pulse beyond the individual and physiological variations of the normal pulse is a diseased pulse.

(1) *Patterns of the pulse and their clinical significance:*

1) Floating pulse: The pulse can be easily detected with the fingers gently applied to the artery, and the pulsation can not be stopped by heavy pressing. This indicates an external deficient syndrome.

2) Deep pulse: The pulse can be detected merely by heavy pressing. This indicates an internal syndrome, and it is an internal excessive syndrome if the pulse is strong; otherwise it is an internal deficient syndrome.

3) Slow pulse: The pulsation of the artery is less than four beats within the time of one breath of the examiner (less than 60 beats in one minute). This indicates a cold syndrome, and it is an excessive cold syndrome if the pulse is strong; otherwise, it is a deficient cold syndrome.

4) Rapid pulse: The palpation of the artery is more than five beats within the time of one breath of the examiner (more than 90 beats in one minute). This indicates a hot syndrome, and it is an excessive hot syndrome, if the pulse is strong; otherwise, it is a deficient hot syndrome.

5) Full pulse: The artery is very wide and the pulsation is like a turbulent wave, with a big range of pulsation. This indicates excessive heat pathogens in the qi component.

6) Large pulse: The artery is as wide as that of the full pulse, but it is not very turbulent and the range of pulsation is not big. This indicates a progressive deficient syndrome in patients with excessive pathogens and the struggle between pathogens and

vital energy can be shown by the stoutness of pulsation.

7) Faint pulse: The artery is fine and weak, and the pulsation is feeble, indistinct and can be stopped by heavy pressure. This indicates deficiency of Yin, Yang, qi and blood.

8) Thready pulse: The artery is as fine as a thread, but the pulsation can be easily detected. This indicates diseases caused by dampness pathogens and various wasting diseases due to deficiency of qi and blood.

9) Scattered pulse: This is a floating and scattered pulse without a solid foundation or a regular rhythm. This indicates exhaustion of vital energy.

10) Feeble pulse: The pulsation at all three portions is feeble and void to the fingers. This indicates a deficient syndrome.

11) Forceful pulse: The pulsation at all three portions is forceful to either gentle or heavy pressing. This indicates an excessive syndrome.

12) Slippery pulse: The pulsation produced by smooth flow of blood in the artery may give a sensation like beads rolling on a plate. This indicates diseases caused by phlegm and rheum, stagnated food or excessive heat pathogens.

13) Uneven pulse: The pulsation comes and goes raggedly, with a joggling sensation, like scratching bamboo with a knife. This indicates loss of essence, depletion of blood, stagnation of qi and blood, and accumulation of phlegm or food.

14) Long pulse: The pulsating artery is longer than the width of three palpating fingers. This indicates excessiveness of liver Yang and endogeneous heat pathogens.

15) Short pulse: The pulsating artery is shorter than the width of three palpating fingers. This indicates stagnation of qi if the pulse is strong; and indicates depletion of qi if the pulse is weak.

16) Stringy pulse: The long and straight artery produces a sensation to the fingers like the string of a musical instrument. This indicates malaria, diseases with pain, diseases caused by phlegm and rheum, and diseases of the liver and gall bladder.

17) Hollow pulse: The pulse is floating, large and hollow, like a piece of green onion leaf. This indicates loss of blood and depletion of Yin.

18) Tense pulse: The artery is as tight as a piece of stretched cord. This indicates a cold syndrome, diseases with pain or stagnation of food.

19) Moderate pulse: The pulsation of the artery is four beats within one breath of the examiner. This indicates deficiency of the spleen and stomach, and diseases caused by dampness pathogens.

20) Leather pulse: The pulse is floating to conduct pulsation and to convey a tough sensation to the palpating fingers, like touching the leather surface of a drum, although it is hollow inside. This indicates loss of blood or essence, incomplete delivery of fetus and dribbling discharge of vaginal blood.

21) Firm pulse: The pulse is forceful, large, stringy and long in nature. This indicates an internal excessive cold syndrome, hernia or tumor in the abdomen.

22) Weak pulse: This is a deep, soft and thready pulse, and indicates deficiency of qi and blood.

23) Soft pulse: This is a floating, thready and soft pulse, and indicates various deficient syndromes or diseases caused by dampness pathogens.

24) Hidden pulse: This is a very deep pulse faintly detectable after the fingers are deeply pressed to reach the bone. This indicates syncope, diseases with severe pain or blockage by pathogens.

25) Tremulous pulse: This is a forceful, rapid and slippery pulse, like a tremulous bean and indicates pain and fright.

26) Fast pulse: This is a rapid pulse with irregular beats and indicates an excessive heat syndrome due to excessive Yang pathogens, stagnation of qi, blood, phlegm, rheum and food, or diseases with pain and swelling.

27) Knotted pulse: This is a slow pulse with irregular beats and indicates accumulation of excessive Yin pathogens, such as cold phlegm or stagnated blood producing masses in the abdomen.

28) Intermittent pulse: This is a slow pulse with regular beats, and indicates exhaustion of qi of the internal organs, wind syndrome, and diseases with pain, fright and external trauma.

29) Swift pulse: This is a very rapid pulse with a frequency of seven to eight beats within a regular breath of the examiner, and indicates depletion of Yang, Yin and vital energy.

(2) *Pulse diagnosis performed by patients upon themselves*:

The pulse is a mirror showing the condition of the heart, and in normal adults the pulse beats are regular and within a range of 60-100 times per minute. Pulsation less than 60 times per minute is known as bradycardia, and the irregular pulsation with dropped beats is called premature beat.

Pathological tachycardia may appear in patients with fever, anemia, pain, cardiac insufficiency, hyperthyroidism, myocarditis, rheumatic fever or pulmonary heart disease; and an irregular pulse with alternation of strong and weak beats may appear in patients of hypertension and arteriosclerotic heart disease, with damage to the myocardium.

The pulsation can be detected by the patients themselves by one of the following methods:

1) Direct palpation over the heart on the left chest by the palm;

2) Palpation on the radial artery by the fingers; and

3) Palpation on the superficial temporal artery in front of the ear by the fingers.

II. Bodily Pain and Self-diagnosis of Diseases

Pain is a common subjective symptom, and it can be divided into headache, pain in the chest and flank, stomachache, abdominal pain, lumbago and pain in the muscles and joints, depending on its location.

The pain may be caused by external wind, cold, summer heat, dampness, dryness and fire pathogens, blocking the meridians and interfering with the transportation of Ying (nutrient) and Wei (defensive energy); by emotional disturbance causing stagnation of qi and blood in internal organs; or by depletion of qi and blood in internal organs and emptiness of blood vessels. In general, distending pain is due to stagnation of qi; pricking pain is due to stagnation of blood; pain with heaviness is caused by dampness pathogens; cold pain with spasms is caused by cold pathogens; burning pain is caused by excessive fire pathogens; lingering pain or pain with an empty sensation and reducible by pressure is a symptom of deficient syndrome; and severe pain or distending pain exacerbated by pressure is a symptom of excessive syndrome.

1. Headache and diagnosis of diseases:

Headache is a common symptom occurring in many diseases

caused by external pathogens, injury to the internal organs or upward attack of endogenous pathogens.

1) Headache in patients with pain in the neck and back exacerbated by coldness, chills induced by wind or cold, soreness and pain in the joints, white thin tongue coating, and floating and tense pulse is due to attack of external wind-cold pathogens, because it may be accumulated to cause stagnation of qi and blood and to block blood vessels.

2) Headache in patients with chills induced by wind, fever, flushed face and ears, thirst with desire to drink water, yellow thin tongue coating, and floating and rapid pulse is due to attack of external wind-heat pathogens, because it can ascend to disturb the orifices of the sense organs.

3) Headache like having a piece of cloth wrapped around the head in patients with dizziness, distending and heavy sensation in the head, exacerbation of headache in cloudy and rainy weather, chills, tiredness of the limbs, heaviness of the body, chest distress, poor appetite, white greasy tongue coating and soft moderate pulse is due to attack of external dampness pathogens, because it can obstruct the orifices of the sense organs and block the ascent of clear Yang and descent of turbid Yang.

4) Distending headache in patients with dizziness, tinnitus, dryness in the eyes, mouth and throat, insomnia, poor memory, numbness and tremor of the limbs, red tongue with scanty moisture and stringy thready pulse is due to upward attack of liver Yang to cause accumulation of qi and blood in the head.

5) Distending headache in patients with flushed face and ears, bitter taste in the mouth, pain in the flanks, anger, constipation, discharge of dark urine, red tip and border of the tongue with yellow dry coating, and stringy rapid pulse is due

to upward flaming of liver fire.

6) Headache with empty sensation in patients with vertigo, tinnitus, weakness of the waist and knee, emission of semen, leukorrhagia, red tongue with scanty coating, and deep, thready and weak pulse is due to deficiency of kidney essence producing enough marrow to enrich the brain.

7) Lingering headache exacerbated by tiredness in patients with chills, shortness of breath, tiredness and weakness of the body, low speaking voice, pale tongue and faint weak pulse is due to deficiency of stomach and spleen qi to nourish the orifices of the sense organs.

8) Dull headache in patients with palpitations of the heart, insomnia, numbness of hands and feet, pale complexion, pale lips and tongue and feeble uneven pulse is due to deficiency of blood to nourish the orifices of the sense organs.

9) Intermittent attacks of headache in patients with dizziness, heaviness of the head and body, tiredness of the limbs, nausea, vomiting of phlegm and rheum, annoyance, white greasy coating and stringy slippery pulse is due to accumulation of turbid phlegm to block ascent of clear Yang and obstruct the orifices of the sense organs.

10) Pricking headache with no definite location may come and go for a long time in patients with dark purple tongue scattered with petechiae, and deep stringy or deep uneven pulse. This is due to stagnation of blood in meridians.

11) Unilateral intolerable migraine may come and go for several days. This is due to transformation of heat pathogens in the liver into phlegm to block the meridians.

12) Tolerable distending headache in patients with swollen head and eyes, blisters on the face, fever, cough, thirst, dryness in the throat, chest distress, yellow greasy tongue coating and

stringy rapid pulse is called Datou Wen (an infectious disease with a swollen head). This is due to upward accumulation of toxic heat pathogens to block meridians.

13) Migraine is a vascular headache, more common in women with a family history of this complaint. Headache may repeatedly appear several times before and after menstruation from adolescence. Before the onset of severe pain on one side of the head and vomiting, the patient may have a prodromal symptom of blurred vision with sparks or bright rings in front of the eyes.

14) Tonic headache is a common type of headache which may occur in 90% of patients with headache. It is a persistent distending pain like wearing a tight cap, and the patients may also suffer from unstable sleep, poor memory, poor concentration, increase of muscular tension, and tenderness in the neck and temporal region.

15) Headache in patients of brain tumor usually appears in the morning, with the severity gradually increasing throughout the day. Headache may be exacerbated by coughing and bending over, and the patients may also suffer from nausea, vomiting, impairment of vision, paralysis of the limbs and epilepsy.

16) Rhinogenous headache caused by parasinusitis may regularly appear in the morning and afternoon, and the patients may have a history of nasal obstruction and passage of purulent nasal discharge, with tenderness detectable over the nose bridge and maxillary sinuses.

17) Paroxymal drilling pain in the occipital region and apparent tenderness at the Fengchi (GB 20) acupoint (foramen of the greater occipital nerve) may appear in patients of greater occipital neuralgia, and with a history of common cold and

spondylopathy.

18) Pain over the superciliary arch, exacerbated by lowering the head, and tenderness at the medial end of this arch may appear in patients of supraorbital neuralgia caused by common cold.

19) Headache epilepsia in children unrelievable by drugs may suddenly appear and disappear, but the sleepiness is retained after the relief of the headache.

20) Temporal arteritis migraine in aged people may cause fever and severe pulsating pain in the temporal region, exacerbated by lying flat and reducible by pressing the carotid artery of the same side. The involved temporal artery is bulging and tender.

2. Pain in the chest and flank, and diagnosis of diseases:

The chest is called Shangjiao (upper energizer) in traditional Chinese medicine, with the heart and lungs contained in it, and the flank is the lateral wall of the chest below the axillary pit with the liver and gallbladder underneath the right flank. Therefore, pain in chest and flank is closely related to diseases of heart, lungs, liver and gallbladder.

1) Chest pain radiating to the back and exacerbated by coldness in patients with palpitations of the heart, shortness of breath, cough, asthma, pale complexion, cold limbs, white tongue coating and deep slow pulse is Bi-syndrome of the chest caused by deficiency of Yang and blockage of Yang from circulating in the chest due to invasion of external cold pathogens.

2) Distending chest pain radiating to the back in patients with asthma, cough and expectoration of sputum, white greasy tongue coating and moderate slippery or stringy slippery pulse is caused by accumulation of phlegm and dampness to block

the normal circulation of Yang qi in the chest.

3) Intermittent pain in thef chest and flanks in patients with chest distress, impatience, anger, bitter taste in the mouth, poor appetite, or palpitations of the heart and shortness of breath, white thin tongue coating and stringy pulse is caused by stagnation of qi in the chest and poor circulation of qi in meridians.

4) Pricking pain at a fixed location of the chest in patients with chest distress, mass beneath the flank, dark purple tongue and uneven pulse is caused by blood stasis in meridians blocking the circulation of qi and blood.

5) Dull pain in the left chest over a long period of time in patients with palpitations of the heart, shortness of breath, insomnia, pale tender tongue and small, weak or knotted and intermittent pulse is caused by deficiency of heart qi and blockage of circulation of qi and blood.

6) Chest pain in patients with dry cough and scanty sputum or without sputum, hemoptysis or blood mixed in sputum, tidal fever, flushed cheekbones, sleep sweats, red tip of tongue and thready rapid pulse is caused by deficiency of lung Yin and burning injury of blood vessels in the lungs by endogenous deficient heat pathogens.

7) Lingering dull pain in the flanks in patients with dizziness, vertigo, hot sensation in the heart, palms and soles of the feet, weakness of the body, dryness in the eyes, red tongue with scanty coating and thready rapid pulse is caused by deficiency of liver Yin to nourish meridians and blood vessels, and scorching of deficient fire pathogens.

8) Chest pain in patients with cough, fever, extreme thirst, spitting of foul sputum or pus and blood, red tongue with yellow coating and slippery rapid pulse is caused by accumulation of toxic heat pathogens in the lungs blocking the blood

vessels.

9) Distending chest pain, exacerbated by cough and spitting of sputum in patients with bulging intercostal spaces, difficulty turning over in bed, white tongue coating and deep stringy pulse is caused by Xuanyin (pleural effusion) due to accumulation of rheum in the chest, blockage of blood vessels and impairment of circulation of qi.

3. Epigastric pain and diagnosis of diseases:

Epigastric pain is also called stomachache, and is caused by improper diet, intake of cold and uncooked food, anxiety and anger, producing blockage of qi.

1) Epigastric pain relievable by hotness in patients with vomiting of clear fluid, extreme coldness of the limbs, bluish white complexion, pale tongue, white thin coating and deep slow pulse is caused by accumulation of cold pathogens in the epigastric region, spasms of the stomach and blockage of stomach qi.

2) Burning epigastric pain in patients with dryness of the mouth and desire to drink cold water, constipation, discharge of dark urine, red tongue and slippery rapid pulse is caused by accumulation of excessive heat pathogens in the stomach and disturbance of circulation of qi.

3) Dull epigastric pain, more remarkable in an empty stomach and relievable after a meal in patients with preference for warmth and pressure applied to the stomach, expectoration of clear fluid, tiredness and weakness of the body, pale complexion, pale tongue with scanty coating and thready weak pulse is caused by deficiency of stomach qi, impairment of the transporting function of the stomach and disturbance of metabolism of body fluid.

4) Lingering dull epigastric pain and hot sensation in patients with poor appetite, fullness in the stomach after a meal, dryness of the lips and tongue, slight thirst, hotness in the heart, palms and soles of the feet, constipation, red tongue and thready rapid pulse is caused by deficiency of stomach Yin and body fluid to moisten the stomach.

5) Distending epigastric pain radiating to the flank region, exacerbated by pressing and relievable after breaking wind in patients with belching, regurgitation of sour fluid, poor appetite, white thin tongue coating and stringy slippery pulse is caused by stagnation of qi and blockage of meridians.

6) Fixed pricking epigastric pain exacerbated by intake of food and pressing on the stomach in patients with tarry stool, bluish tongue with ecchymoses and deep uneven pulse is caused by blood stasis and blockage of blood vessels.

7) Distending epigastric pain aggravated by pressing on the stomach in patients with nausea, vomiting, regurgitation of sour and foul substance, poor appetite, foul stool difficult to be completely voided, yellow greasy or mixed yellow and white tongue coating and forceful slippery pulse is caused by accumulation of food in the stomach, disturbance of circulation of qi and impairment of downward transportation of stomach qi.

4. Abdominal pain and diagnosis of diseases:

Abdominal pain indicates a pain below the epigastric region and above the pubic symphysis, and it is divided into upper, middle and lower abdominal pain. The liver, gallbladder, spleen, kidneys, colon, small intestine, urinary bladder and uterus are all contained in the abdomen, and the abdominal pain may be caused by invasion of external pathogens, injury to the internal organs, blockage of circulation of qi and blood or deficiency of qi and blood to warm and nourish the internal organs.

1) Continuous severe spastic abdominal pain with tenderness relievable by hotness in patients with a gurgling sound in the intestines, diarrhea, white thin tongue coating and deep tense pulse is caused by accumulation of cold pathogens in the abdomen and blockage of circulation of qi.

2) Burning and distending abdominal pain with tenderness in patients with preference for coldness and aversion to heat, thirst, constipation, red tongue with a yellow coating and slippery rapid pulse is caused by accumulation of fire and heat pathogens, and blockage of circulation of qi.

3) Distending pain wandering around the abdomen without fixed location but relievable after breaking wind in patients with poor appetite, discomfort after meals, white thin coating and stringy slippery pulse is caused by stagnation of qi and blood, and blockage of blood vessels.

4) Abdominal pain with tenderness or mass at a fixed location and worse at night in patients with bluish tongue scattered with ecchymoses, and deep uneven pulse is caused by stagnation of blood and blockage of circulation of qi.

5) Intermittent pain around the umbilicus with fusiform mass appearing and disappearing from time to time in patients with thin body, sallow complexion, teeth-grinding, milia on the inner surface of the lips and deep tense pulse during attack of abdominal pain is caused by ascaris stimulating the intestines and blocking the circulation of qi.

6) Sudden onset of intolerable colic pain in the right upper quadrant of the abdomen in patients with pale complexion, sweating, cold limbs, nausea, vomiting of vomitus with ascaris, normal tongue and deep tense pulse is caused by ascaris in the

194

biliary tract.

7) Relaptic dull abdominal pain with preference for warmth and pressure applied over the abdomen in patients with mental and physical tiredness, cold limbs, loose stool, pale tongue with a white coating and deep, thready and weak pulse is caused by deficiency of Yang and failure to produce qi due to deficient cold pathogens.

8) Abdominal pain with passage of stool mixed with red blood and white pus, tenesmus, burning sensation in the anus, discharge of small amounts of dark urine, red tongue, yellow greasy pulse and slippery rapid pulse is caused by dysentery due to accumulation of damp-heat pathogens in the intestines and blockage of transportation of qi.

9) Spastic pain in the right lower quadrant with tenderness and mass in patients with nausea, vomiting, difficulty in flexing and extending the right leg, yellow greasy tongue coating and stringy rapid pulse is caused by intestinal abscess due to accumulation of heat pathogens in the intestines and blockage of circulation of qi.

Dysmenorrhea in women, with severe pain in lower abdomen and waist, pale complexion, cold sweating, cold limbs, nausea and vomiting is caused by disturbance of Chòngmai (thoroughfare vessel) and Renmai (conceptional vessel), and impairment of circulation of qi and blood through meridians.

5. Pain in the muscles and joints and diagnosis of diseases:

Pain in the muscles and joints is known as Bi-syndrome in traditional Chinese medicine, and it is caused by attack of external wind, cold, dampness and heat pathogens blocking circulation of qi and blood through the meridians.

1) Wandering arthralgia of the upper limbs with limitation

of movement of joints in patients of wind Bi-syndrome is caused by attack of wind pathogens, because the wind is constantly changing in intensity and direction.

2) Severe arthralgia at a definite location with limitation of movement, preference for heat, fear of cold, white tongue coating and stringy and tense pulse is cold Bi-syndrome caused by attack of cold pathogens producing stagnation of qi and blood in the meridians.

3) Aching pain in the muscles and joints in fixed areas of the waist, back and lower limbs with local heaviness, numbness and swelling, white greasy tongue coating and soft moderate pulse is dampness Bi-syndrome. The dampness pathogens are turbid, heavy, sticky and greasy in nature, and can accumulate in joints, blocking circulation of qi.

4) Burning arthralgia with redness, swelling and hot feeling over a joint relievable by coldness in patients with fever, annoyance, thirst, yellow tongue coating and slippery rapid pulse is hot Bi-syndrome caused by attack of heat pathogens scorching muscles and joints and producing an accumulation of qi and blood, which can be transformed into heat pathogens again after a long time.

5) Aching pain in muscles and joints in patients with spasms in the muscles and blood vessels, palpitations of the heart, shortness of breath, spontaneous sweating, general weakness, sallow complexion, pale tongue and weak pulse is Bi-syndrome due to deficiency of qi and blood and blockage of the meridians by wind, cold and dampness pathogenss for a long time.

6) Fixed pricking pain in the joints of the limbs, worse at night in patients with swollen and deformed joints, difficulty in extending and flexing the joints, hotness in the heart, palms

and soles of the feet, dark purple skin, engorged blood vessels, bluish tongue with petechiae and stringy or deep uneven pulse is Bi-syndrome caused by blood stasis due to impairment of circulation of qi and blood, and blockage of qi and blood in blood vessels.

III. Self-diagnosis of Diseases

1. Ten criteria of a healthy body and mind:

1) Healthy people should be full of physical and mental energy so that they can carry out their work and daily life in a leisurely way and without suffering.

2) They always keep an optimistic view and active attitude when carrying out their tasks no matter how difficult or tedious these are.

3) They can rest and sleep well.

4) They have a good adaptibility to fit in with change of environment.

5) They have a good bodily resistance to the common cold and ordinary infectious diseases.

6) They have the proper weight and height, and always keep an adequate standing posture, with the head, arms and hips in a coordinated position.

7) Their eyes are bright, without inflammation, and the reflex of the pupils is active.

8) The teeth are clean, without caries or pain; and the gums are normal in color, without bleeding.

9) The hair is sleek and glossy, without dandruff.

10) They can walk with brisk steps, and the skin and muscles are very elastic.

2. Self-diagnosis of overfatigue: Overfatigue may occur in the following situations:

1) The work load is doubled.

2) The work is continued over 10 hours every day.

3) The work is irregularly arranged and often continued late into the night.

4) Holidays are often given up for work over a long period of time.

5) Frequent business trips without enough rest and sleep at home.

6) Bad relationships with colleagues.

7) Running or working in a badly managed organization, especially when the person is responsible for poor management.

8) Smoking over 30 cigarettes a day.

9) Alcohol consumed daily for several months.

10) Drinking five cups of coffee every day for over one year.

11) The time and amount of meals are uncertain and the food contains too much animal fat.

12) Returning home after 10 pm every night for several months.

13) Sweating without physical exertion over a long period of time.

14) Believing oneself to be healthy, and not consulting a doctor for two to three years.

15) Suffering from hypertension, heart disease or diabetes mellitus.

16) Marked increase or decrease of body weight.

17) Soreness and weakness in the body.

18) Easily becoming tired and easily becoming drunk after taking only a small amount of alcohol.

19) Frequent severe headaches or pain and distress in the chest.

20) The memory suddenly becomes poor.

21) Sudden appearance of senility.

If nine of the above 21 criteria are positive a person should immediately consult a doctor.

3. Warning signs of diseases:

1) Decline in body resistance.

2) Tiring easily.

3) Lack of stamina to pursue an activity and easily feeling impatient.

4) Too weak to go upstairs or downstairs.

5) Sluggish in making a response in conversation and forgetful.

6) Disinclined to work.

7) Susceptible to common cold, and refractory to treatment.

8) Poor appetite.

9) Constantly feeling cold in the waist and legs.

10) Sallow complexion and weak body.

11) Constantly late in rising.

12) Soreness of the shoulders and headache.

13) Soreness and pain in the waist and knees.

14) Constantly feeling tired and sleepy.

15) Easily intoxicated.

16) Sudden reduction of tolerance for alcohol.

17) Sore and aching back and waist after light physical exertion.

18) Discomfort in the stomach.

19) Extraordinary tiredness after delivery of a baby.

20) Hoarse voice.

21) Constantly feeling thirsty at night, and wanting to drink much water.

22) Highly irritable without apparent reason.

23) Soreness in the chest and shortness of breath while walking.

24) The sudden change of defecation habit.

25) The increase of frequency of urination, with an increase of urine amount.

26) Numbness in the hands and feet.

27) Irregular menstruation and dysmenorrhea.

28) Dizziness and vertigo when standing up.

29) Tinnitus and insomnia.

30) Anxiety.

31) The skin becomes rough and lusterless.

32) A blocked sensation in the pharynx when swallowing food.

A person with any one of the above phenomena should consult a doctor.

4. Self-diagnosis of avitaminosis:

1) Avitaminosis A: The patient may suffer from dry and rough skin, dryness in the eyes, photophobia, lachrymation, progressive blurred vision and susceptibility to infection of the respiratory tract.

2) Avitaminosis B1: The patient may suffer from indigestion, sallow complexion, numbness of the hands and feet, multiple neuritis and beriberi.

3) Avitaminosis B3: The patient may suffer from a foul smell from mouth, insomnia, headache and mental tiredness.

4) Avitaminosis B12: The patient may suffer from pale skin, sparse hair, lassitude, poor appetite, vomiting and diarrhea.

5) Avitaminosis C: The patient may suffer from swelling of purple gums, bleeding tendency of conjunctiva and skin and stubborn wound.

6) Avitaminosis D: The patient may suffer from sweating, rickets in children and osteomalacia in adults.

7) Avataminosis E: The patient may suffer from sweating, split hair and mental nervousness.

5. Warning signs of cancer:

(1) *There are eight warnings of cancer proposed by the World Health Organization (WHO)*:

1) Palpable hard nodules or masses in the breast or on the skin and tongue.

2) Change of nature and color of nevi and warts.

3) Persistent indigestion.

4) Persistent hoarseness of voice, dry cough or dysphagia.

5) Profuse menstrual bleeding or vaginal bleeding not related to menstruation.

6) Bleeding from the ear, nose, urinary bladder or intestines without apparent cause.

7) Stubborn wound which does not heal over a long period of time or irresolvable swelling.

8) Unreasonable loss of body weight.

(2) *Warning signs of common cancers in China*:

1) Palpable and irresolvable masses in the breast or on the skin, tongue or other parts of the body.

2) Rapid change of color and size of warts and nevi, with itching, exudate, ulceration or bleeding.

3) Persistent indigestion.

4) Dysphagia, pain and distress behind the sternum, sensation of a foreign body in the stomach or pain in the upper abdomen.

5) Tinnitus, impairment of hearing, nasal obstruction, nasal bleeding, bloody nasal discharge, headache and masses in the neck region.

6) Irregular menstrual bleeding, irregular vaginal bleeding after menopause or not related to menstruation or sexual intercourse bleeding.

7) Persistent hoarseness of the voice, dry cough and blood in sputum.

8) Blood and mucus in stool and constant alternation of diarrhea and constipation or hematuria without apparent cause.

9) Stubborn wound or ulcer difficult to heal over a long period of time and swelling difficult to resolve.

10) Loss of body weight without apparent cause.

6. Self-diagnosis of lung cancer:

1) Cough: Stimulating cough after physical effort without sputum or with scanty sputum.

2) Blood in sputum: Fresh blood streaks are present in white sticky sputum and the condition is refractory to treatment.

3) Pain and distress in the chest: At the early stage, the chest pain and distress is intermittent. Then the pain turns continuous, distending, depressing and pricking in nature, and it may be exacerbated by physical exertion, change of posture, deep breath and cough.

4) Shortness of breath: People normally in good health may suddenly develop shortness of breath during light physical effort.

5) General symptoms: The patient may also suffer from

fever, weakness, lassitude and hoarseness of the voice.

6) The patient may have arthralgia and black spots along creases of the skin, and male patients may have hyperplasia of the breasts. Tender clubbed fingers and toes may appear and quickly grow in size with a red inflammatory zone of skin along the roots of the nails.

7. Self-diagnosis of cancer of testis:

1) A painless mass appears in the testis and produces a heavy sensation to patients in a standing posture.

2) The testis is diffusely increased in size.

3) The testis is increased in size with a nodular shape, uneven consistency and tenderness to palpation.

4) A mass in the lower abdomen or inguinal region may appear in patients with undescended testis.

5) The skin of the scrotum may become smooth.

8. Important symptoms of AIDS:

1) Extreme weakness of the whole body, worse in the morning.

2) Profuse sweating at night as well as during the day.

3) Impairment of digestion, poor appetite and rapid loss of body weight of about eight kg in one month.

4) Enteritis with frequent diarrhea.

5) Enlargement of the lymph nodes in the neck, behind the ear, below the shoulder and in the inguinal groove.

6) Fever, injury to the skin, mucosa in the oral cavity and white furry patches on the tongue.

7) Vesicles and various rashes on the skin.

AIDS can be divided into three stages:

(1) The incubation period lasts from a few months to several years.

(2) The second stage, with symptoms of the lymphatic system, may last for one or more years.

(3) In the third stage, the patient may suffer from severe anemia and leukocytopenia, especially lymphocytopenia.

9. Clinical manifestations of severe febrile diseases:

1) Cool body and limbs and overfatigue after sudden reduction of high fever.

2) Persistent high fever.

3) High fever in bedridden patients.

4) Fever in patients with emaciation of the body.

5) Fever in patients with sores on the body.

6) Fever in patients with dyspnea.

7) Fever in patients with reduced discharge of urine.

8) Fever in patients with sallow complexion.

9) Fever in patients with mental confusion.

10) Fever in patients with convulsions.

10. Prodromal symptoms of apoplexy (stroke):

1) Sudden onset of numbness of one arm, one leg or one side of the face.

2) Suddenly difficulty in speaking.

3) Sudden loss of vision for a few seconds to several minutes.

4) Vertigo, unsteady gait or sudden falling down.

5) Extraordinarily severe headache, drowsiness, nausea and vomiting.

6) Sudden change of personality, poor judgment and poor memory.

11. Self-diagnosis of ascariasis in young children:

1) Frequent abdominal pain usually occurring around the umbilicus without apparent cause.

2) Repeated appearance of urticaria without apparent inducing factors.

3) Mental nervousness and high irritability in short durations during the day and teeth-grinding at night.

4) Red round papules with regular borders scattered on the protruded tongue.

5) Greyish white pinpoint granules densely scattered along the borders of the gums.

6) Blue triangular, round or semilunar spots scattered on the sclera of the eyes.

7) White round skin lesions in the size of the finger pad, with fine scales on the face.

8) Gradual emaciation of the body in spite of a good appetite in babies.

9) Poor mental concentration.

12. Self-diagnosis of arteriosclerosis:

1) Difficulty in remembering the names of people, figures and the date.

2) Dizziness and headache varying in intensity from time to time.

3) Tremor of the hand, especially apparent when holding chopsticks to pick up food or holding a pen to write.

4) Change of personality with high irritability, unstable emotions, sudden change of joy, anger, sadness and happiness, and speaking nonsense.

5) Presence of formication over local skin.

6) Slow motion of the limbs and body, and mental retarda-

tion.

13. Early symptoms of liver diseases:

1) Disorder of digestion without apparent inducing factors, such as remarkable reduction of food intake by 2/3 of the normal amount, nausea, vomiting, aversion to oily food, constipation or diarrhea.

2) Unstable emotions, change of personality from cheerfulness to sadness or from quietness to restlessness, and impairment of sleep.

3) Apparent loss of physical energy, general tiredness and weakness, soreness in the limbs not relievable by rest, poor memory, low working efficiency, poor mental concentration and liability to make mistakes.

4) Jaundice of the skin and eyes, and discharge of yellow urine like dark tea may appear in patients without other discomforts; but jaundice may be absent in patients with fever, discomfort in the upper abdomen and the above symptoms at the early stage of liver diseases.

14. Prevention of cancers:

1) Have a wide variety of food and taste.

2) Do not keep the same regimen of diet or take the same drug for a long time.

3) Avoid very heavy or oily meals.

4) Do not consume alcohol to excess.

5) Do not smoke.

6) Take an adequate dosage of vitamins A, C and E and eat more green vegetables, fruits and food rich in vitamins.

7) Avoid food which is too salty or too hot.

8) Avoid burnt food.

9) Avoid rotten food.

10) Avoid strong sunlight.

11) Avoid overfatigue.

12) Bathe frequently.

15. Self-diagnosis of neurasthenia:

1) The patient may often have palpitations of the heart and distress in the chest.

2) After a busy day's work, the patient indulges in excessive smoking and drinking rather than taking a rest, resulting in a disturbed mood, insomnia and nightmares.

3) The patient may be greatly depressed by some minor discomfort and worried about suffering from some serious diseases, although the suspicion has already been disproved by a thorough medical examination.

4) The patient is argumentative at home, although regarded as an excellent worker.

5) The patient drinks alcohol with increasing tolerance, and does not mind its harmfulness.

6) The patient has no appetite for food although feeling hungry; and suffers from impotence despite sexual desire.

7) The patient may have an odd personality and a bad relationship with colleagues, often muttering to himself or herself.

8) The patient can not accept corrections, proposals or appraisals from colleagues, and are enraged by different opinions and criticism.

9) The patient reads books for preserving health without clear purpose and can not persistently follow the guidance in such books.

10) The patient gets very impatient during rush hours, quite different from the previous mood.

11) The patient becomes too tired to carry on doing accustomed physical exercise.

12) The patient loses interest in reading books, newspaper and magazines.

图书在版编目（CIP）数据

察颜观色测百病：英文 / 刘帮明主编.
一北京：外文出版社，2002
ISBN 7-119-02028-5
I. 察…　II. 刘…　III.疾病－望诊（中医）－英文
IV. R24 1. 2
中国版本图书馆 CIP 数据核字（98）第 02584 号

责任编辑	余冰清
封面设计	蔡　荣
插图绘制	李士仪
印刷监制	冯　浩

外文出版社网址：
　http://www.flp.com.cn
外文出版社电子信箱：
　info@flp.com.cn
　sales@flp.com.cn

察颜观色测百病

刘帮明　主编

*

©外文出版社
外文出版社出版
（中国北京百万庄大街 24 号）
邮政编码　100037
三河市实验小学印刷厂印刷
中国国际图书贸易总公司发行
（中国北京车公庄西路 35 号）
北京邮政信箱第 399 号　邮政编码　100044
2002 年(大 32 开)第 1 版
2002 年第 1 版第 1 次印刷
（英）
ISBN 7-119-02028-5/R.148(外)
03000(平)
14-E-3182 P